Beating the Heat

Essential Strategies to Protect Children's Lives in Hot Weather

Brenda F. Dozier

Gratitude

Dear, Reader!

Beating the Heat: Essential Strategies to Protect Children's Lives in Hot Weather is a book that we are grateful you have chosen to read. The fact that you have chosen to purchase this book demonstrates that you are dedicated to ensuring the health and happiness of the children in your life. It is possible that your proactive attitude could make all the difference in a world where temperatures are rising and the risks of heat-related illnesses are becoming more widespread.

Knowing that every child needs to be protected from the harmful effects of high heat, this book was produced with a profound sense of responsibility and compassion for the children who need protection. It does not matter if you are a parent, a caregiver, a teacher, or just someone concerned about the well-being of children; the role that you play in putting the concepts and facts that are presented in these pages into practice is extremely valuable.

It is an honor that you have decided to spend some of your time with the words and counsel that are provided in this book. I am aware that your time is valuable, and thanks for your consideration. Your unwavering commitment to acquiring and implementing these tactics is not only admirable, but it is also very necessary to make the atmosphere in which the children you care about are raised safer.

I would like you to know that your support is really important to me. Your dedication to this cause, regardless of whether you are a parent, caregiver, educator, or community leader, enhances our collective capacity to safeguard those who are the most vulnerable among us. If this book helps even one youngster avoid the hazards of heat-related illnesses, then our efforts together have made a difference.

Your devotion to understanding and adopting these vital measures not only helps protect the children in your care but also contributes to a greater culture of awareness and prevention. By taking these steps, you are playing a critical part in a bigger campaign to keep our communities safe and healthy.

Thank you for being a part of this vital mission. Your actions today will surely make a difference in the lives of many tomorrows. Stay cautious, stay aware, and continue to safeguard those who depend on you the most.

With heartfelt thanks,

Brenda F. Dozier

Table of Contents

Because of the persistent rise in temperatures, it is becoming increasingly difficult to disregard the risks associated with hot weather. When it comes to children, the danger is considerably higher. Because their bodies are still developing and significantly more susceptible to damage than those of adults, they face a unique set of obstacles when they are subjected to elevated temperatures. On the other hand, the severity of these dangers is frequently overestimated, which leaves children in a precarious position where they are vulnerable to the potentially fatal effects of heat-related disorders. The repercussions can be immediate, severe, and terrible, and unfortunately, they are frequently avoidable too.

Rather than merely being a guide, "Beating the Heat: Essential Strategies to Protect Children's Lives in Hot Weather" is more of a rallying cry for people to take action. To ensure that children are safe, healthy, and protected during the sweltering days of summer and beyond, this book is intended for parents, caregivers, teachers, and members of the community who want to make sure that children are safeguarded. On these pages, you will find guidance from professionals, helpful hints, and essential information that could be the deciding factor in whether or not you live or die. The purpose of this is not to scare you; rather, it is to provide you with the knowledge and tools necessary to prevent inconceivable circumstances.

The necessity for vigilance is increasing in tandem with the rise in global temperatures. Heat-related ailments, including dehydration, heat exhaustion, and heatstroke, are genuine hazards, and they don't discriminate. Children from all walks of life, whether playing at the park, attending summer camp, or simply spending time at home, can rapidly find themselves in danger if the proper precautions aren't taken. But here's the good news: most heat-related catastrophes are fully preventable with the correct awareness and action.

In a world where we can't always control the climate, we can control how we respond to it. "Beating the Heat" is your comprehensive reference, packed with important tips to keep your children safe when the temperature soars. You'll learn how to spot the early warning symptoms of heat-related illnesses, implement effective preventive measures, and respond rapidly in crises. You'll also discover the value of community support, how to lobby for safer situations, and why teaching children themselves is a critical step in protecting them.

The protection of our children should never be left to chance. As you turn the pages of this book, you'll be taking a proactive step toward safeguarding their health and well-being. This is more than just a read—it's a lifeline for every parent and caregiver who wishes to preserve the most precious and vulnerable among us.

Don't wait for disaster to hit before you take action. Equip yourself with the knowledge and courage to keep your children safe, no matter how high the mercury rises.

"Beating the Heat: Essential Strategies to Protect Children's Lives in Hot Weather" is your guide to ensuring that the children in your care not only survive but develop, even in the face of the most demanding conditions. Let this book be your friend in the fight against heat, since when it comes to the safety of our children, nothing less than complete preparedness will do.

Overview of Heat-Related Risks for Children

The rising temperatures associated with summer months pose considerable hazards to children, who are uniquely exposed to the impacts of intense heat. Heat-related disorders, such as dehydration, heat exhaustion, and heatstroke, are hazardous symptoms that can worsen quickly and lead to long-term health consequences or even death. Unlike adults, children's bodies are not fully mature, making them less efficient in regulating temperature. Their higher metabolic rates, coupled with a greater surface area-to-body weight ratio, mean they absorb heat more quickly and struggle to cool down as effectively. In hot weather, children are also more inclined to engage in physical activity, increasing their risk of overheating. The combination of these variables puts them at a substantially higher risk during periods of intense heat.

Impact of Climate Changing and Rising Global Temperatures

Climate change is driving a continuous increase in global temperatures, leading to more frequent and extreme heatwaves. These heatwaves are not only an annoyance; they are a significant public health danger, particularly for children. As the planet heats, cities and towns around the world are experiencing higher average temperatures, extended periods of intense heat, and a growing number of dangerously hot days each year. The repercussions of climate change extend beyond the heat itself. Changes in weather patterns can lead to droughts, wildfires, and other environmental difficulties that compound the dangers posed by hot weather. In urban locations, the heat island effect—where concrete and asphalt absorb and keep heat—can push temperatures even higher, making it much more difficult for youngsters to find relief. These rising temperatures are a strong signal that aggressive steps are needed to safeguard those most in danger, notably children.

The Importance of Safeguarding Children During Extreme Heat

Protecting children during instances of excessive heat is not just about comfort; it is about preserving their safety and health. Children rely on parents to maintain a safe environment, and during hot weather, this role takes on increased significance. Safeguarding children includes taking proactive actions to prevent heat-related illnesses before they arise. This involves ensuring that children are sufficiently hydrated, limiting their exposure to the sun during the hottest times of the day, and making sure they have access to cool places. It also involves educating youngsters about the necessity of staying cool and recognizing the indications of heat-related sickness. For children with current health concerns, such as asthma or obesity, the dangers are significantly greater, making monitoring all the more vital. The goal is to establish a safe environment where children can continue to enjoy their everyday activities without the worry of heat-related sickness hanging over them.

Why Children Are More Vulnerable to Heat Than Adults

Children's bodies are still growing and developing, which makes them more exposed to the dangers of excessive heat. Their tiny size means they absorb heat more quickly than adults, and their bodies are less efficient at cooling down through perspiration. Children also have a faster metabolic rate, which generates more internal heat. Unlike adults, who may recognize the need to slow down or seek shade when they begin to feel overheated, children are generally less aware of the indicators of heat stress and may continue playing or exerting themselves even when they are dangerously hot. Additionally, young children, particularly infants and toddlers, are unable to express when they are feeling overheated, making it even more crucial for caregivers to watch them regularly. These physiological variations underscore the need for extra care and attention to keep youngsters safe during hot weather.

Understanding these concerns is the first step in safeguarding children from the perils of severe heat. It is vital to remember that what could be a small inconvenience for an adult can suddenly become a life-threatening issue for a child. As temperatures continue to climb internationally, ensuring that children are protected from the negative impacts of heat is more critical than ever.

Highlight the risks associated with high temperatures and climate change.

The rise of high temperatures owing to climate change entails major dangers that are especially alarming for vulnerable populations, including children. Prolonged exposure to excessive heat can lead to a range of health concerns, from minor discomfort to severe, life-threatening diseases. Heat exhaustion and heatstroke are two of the most serious effects, with the latter being a medical emergency that can cause lasting damage to the brain and other essential organs if not treated swiftly. In addition to these acute threats, there are longer-term consequences. Chronic exposure to high temperatures has been associated with respiratory troubles, cardiovascular problems, and the exacerbation of existing health concerns such as asthma. The cumulative consequences of climate change, particularly more frequent and intense heat waves, raise the likelihood of these health concerns. Moreover, high heat can impair key services, like electricity and water supply, further exacerbating the difficulty of keeping children safe during hot weather.

The Importance of Awareness and Proactive Measures

Awareness is the first line of defense in safeguarding children from the dangers of severe heat. Understanding the dangers and identifying the indicators of heat-related illnesses is critical for parents, caregivers, and community members. Without awareness, the risk can go unknown until it is too late. Proactive measures are equally vital; they are the efforts performed to prevent heat-related problems before they emerge. This includes basic but effective techniques like ensuring children stay hydrated, dressing them in lightweight, breathable clothing, and minimizing outside activity during high-heat hours. Creating a cool environment at home and understanding when to seek medical assistance are also crucial components of a preventative strategy. Educating youngsters about the necessity of staying cool and detecting when they are feeling too hot is another crucial step. With understanding and proactive actions, many of the problems connected with excessive heat can be reduced, sparing children from needless harm.

Thesis Statement

With the correct methods, parents and caregivers can help keep children safe and healthy during hot weather. This requires a combination of awareness, education, and action. By knowing the hazards posed by high temperatures and taking simple, yet effective steps, adults can greatly minimize the chance of heat-related diseases in children. The obligation rests in ensuring that children are not only comfortable but also safe from the potentially lethal effects of severe heat. The goal is to create an environment where children can thrive, even when the temperatures spike, by being well-prepared and aware.

This strategy for protecting children in hot weather emphasizes the significance of preparation and awareness. Parents and caregivers must be prepared with the knowledge and resources necessary to anticipate potential risks and take fast action when needed. This entails remaining educated about weather forecasts, identifying the indications of heat-related stress, and knowing how to respond to crises. It also entails making deliberate judgments about children's activities, ensuring that they are not exposed to unnecessary heat during the hottest portions of the day.

In addition to urgent efforts, long-term planning is vital. This could mean investing in house cooling solutions, such as fans or air conditioning, and ensuring that outdoor play places are shaded and safe. Schools, daycares, and community centers should also be included in these initiatives, creating rules and procedures that prioritize the safety of children during high heat. By establishing community-wide knowledge and response to the dangers of high temperatures, the risk to children can be further mitigated.

At its core, the purpose is to provide a secure atmosphere for children, where they may enjoy their summer days without the fear of heat-related illnesses. This needs a concerted effort from everyone involved in a child's upbringing, from parents and caregivers to educators and community leaders. When these measures are skillfully executed, they create a powerful defense against the risks of severe heat, ensuring that children remain safe, healthy, and protected.

Safeguarding children during hot weather is not simply about reacting to the heat when it gets unbearable—it's about being proactive and prepared, employing informed techniques to prevent harm. The responsibility to safeguard children from the hazards of high temperatures is a common one, requiring awareness, action, and a commitment to their well-being. With the appropriate strategy, parents and caregivers can successfully negotiate the obstacles of hot weather, keeping children safe and ensuring that they can continue to enjoy their activities, even in the heat of summer.

Chapter 1

Understanding Heat-Related Illnesses

Heat-related illnesses are a major and even life-threatening risk, particularly for children. These conditions emerge when the body is unable to cool itself efficiently in hot temperatures. Normally, the body maintains its temperature by perspiration, but under excessive heat, this natural cooling process can become overwhelming. When the body absorbs more heat than it can emit, core temperatures rise, leading to a range of health complications. Understanding the many forms of heat-related illnesses and their symptoms is vital for averting serious complications. Early recognition and timely action can dramatically minimize the likelihood of serious outcomes.

Common Heat-Related Illnesses in Children

Children are more prone to heat-related illnesses because their bodies are still developing and are less effective at controlling temperature. Among the most prevalent heat-related disorders in children are heat exhaustion and heatstroke. These disorders, while related, range in severity and require various approaches to therapy. Both can occur fast and without notice, particularly in circumstances where youngsters are physically active or exposed to direct sunlight for extended periods. It's crucial for parents, caregivers, and educators to be familiar with the indicators of these illnesses and to take early action if symptoms arise.

Heat Exhaustion

Heat exhaustion is a condition that happens when the body loses too much water and salt through excessive perspiration. It is generally triggered by extended exposure to high temperatures, especially when accompanied by physical activity. The symptoms of heat exhaustion include profuse perspiration, weakness, disorientation, nausea, headaches, and muscle cramps. Children experiencing heat exhaustion may also seem pale, feel faint, or have cold, clammy skin. While heat exhaustion is less serious than heatstroke, it can swiftly escalate if not managed. Immediate therapy comprises relocating the kid to a cooler area, urging them to relax, and offering fluids, preferably with electrolytes, to replenish lost salts. Monitoring is vital, as untreated heat exhaustion can develop into heatstroke, which is significantly more hazardous.

Heatstroke

Heatstroke is the utmost form of heat-related disease and constitutes a medical emergency. It occurs when the body's temperature regulating mechanism fails, leading to a rapid and dangerous rise in core body temperature, generally beyond 104°F (40°C). Unlike heat exhaustion, which is characterized by heavy perspiration, heatstroke generally appears with hot, dry skin due to the cessation of sweating. Other symptoms include confusion, changed mental state, convulsions, and loss of consciousness. If left untreated, heatstroke can result in permanent damage to the brain and other essential organs, or even death. Immediate action is essential if heatstroke is suspected. This involves alerting emergency services, relocating the child to a cool environment, and attempting to lower their body temperature by measures such as administering cool water to the skin, utilizing fans, or placing ice packs on vital areas including the neck, armpits, and groin. Quick intervention is crucial to enhancing outcomes and minimizing the risk of long-term health impacts.

Dehydration

Dehydration occurs when the body loses more fluids than it takes in, resulting in an imbalance that can affect key physical functions. In hot weather, children are particularly prone to dehydration because they are more likely to be active outdoors, sweating more and losing fluids rapidly. Dehydration can happen swiftly, especially if a youngster is not drinking enough water or consuming beverages that don't appropriately replenish lost fluids. The illness can range in severity, from moderate cases that induce thirst and dry mouth to more significant cases that lead to dizziness, confusion, and even fainting. In extreme dehydration, the body's ability to regulate temperature weakens, raising the risk of heat-related disorders such as heat exhaustion and heatstroke. It's crucial to urge children to drink water regularly, particularly while they are playing outside or engaged in vigorous activities. Keeping children hydrated is a critical preventative action against the risks of hot weather.

Heat Cramps

Heat cramps are painful muscle spasms that develop as a result of high sweating after severe physical exercise in hot conditions. They are most typically encountered in the belly, arms, and legs, and are a direct consequence of the loss of electrolytes, such as sodium, potassium, and magnesium, through sweat. While heat cramps are normally not life-threatening, they are a symptom that the body is straining to cope with the heat and may be on the verge of more serious conditions like heat exhaustion. Children experiencing heat cramps may feel powerful, involuntary muscle contractions that can be distressing and uncomfortable. Immediate relief often entails ceasing physical activity, relocating to a cooler environment, and consuming fluids that contain electrolytes to replenish the body's salt levels. Stretching the afflicted muscles and massaging the constricted areas might also help ease the discomfort. Preventing heat cramps entails ensuring that youngsters stay hydrated and take breaks during vigorous activities in hot circumstances.

Sunburn and Skin Damage

Sunburn occurs when the skin is exposed to ultraviolet (UV) rays from the sun for an extended period without proper protection. For youngsters, whose skin is more sensitive than that of adults, sunburn can happen fast and inflict substantial pain and damage. Sunburn not only causes acute discomfort, such as redness, swelling, and blistering, but it also raises the risk of long-term skin damage, including accelerated aging and a higher chance of skin cancer. Repeated sunburns throughout youth are particularly worrying, as they can contribute to a higher probability of getting melanoma and other skin malignancies later in life. To protect children against sunburn, it is vital to apply a broad-spectrum sunscreen with an SPF of at least 30 to all exposed skin, reapplying it every two hours or more often if swimming or sweating. Additionally, wearing protective clothing, hats, and sunglasses can help shield the skin from dangerous UV rays. It's crucial to remember that even on cloudy days, UV rays can permeate through the clouds, making sun protection necessary at all times when outdoors.

Signs and Symptoms

Recognizing the signs and symptoms of heat-related disorders is crucial for preventing severe results. Early identification allows for timely intervention, which can prevent the illness from worsening. Common indicators of dehydration include dry mouth, thirst, dark yellow urine, lethargy, and dizziness. As dehydration advances, symptoms may include intense thirst, irritation, confusion, and, in severe cases, fainting or coma. For heat cramps, the major symptom is rapid, painful muscle spasms, generally in the legs, arms, or belly, commonly occurring during or after vigorous physical activity.

In the case of sunburn, the symptoms often include red, sore skin that is warm to the touch, and in more severe cases, blistering and edema. Children may also experience fever, chills, and nausea if the sunburn is significant. Over time, the damaged skin may peel as it heals, which can be unpleasant and raise the risk of infection if not properly cared for.

Heat exhaustion appears with a variety of symptoms, including intense perspiration, weakness, disorientation, nausea, headaches, and muscle cramps. Children may also feel faint, and their skin could appear chilly and damp despite the heat. If heat exhaustion is not addressed, it can escalate to heatstroke, which is characterized by a high body temperature (over 104°F), confusion, fast breathing, and a lack of sweating despite the heated environment. Heatstroke is a medical emergency that requires quick attention to avert serious consequences or death.

Being aware of these signs and symptoms is vital for anyone caring for children in hot weather. Early detection and management can make a major difference in reducing the progression of heat-related diseases and ensuring that children remain safe and well.

Impact of Heat-Related Conditions on Children's Health

Heat-related disorders can have substantial and immediate repercussions on children's health, potentially leading to both acute and long-term consequences. Dehydration, if left untreated, can impair cognitive function, limit physical performance, and, in extreme situations, induce kidney damage and other systemic failures. Heat exhaustion, albeit less severe than heatstroke, can nevertheless cause significant distress, leading to extended weakness, weariness, and, in some cases, hospitalization. If not managed promptly, heat exhaustion can escalate to heatstroke, a life-threatening condition. Heatstroke can cause damage to the brain, heart, kidneys, and muscles, with the possibility of long-term impairments or death. Sunburns, particularly recurrent or severe ones, not only cause acute pain and agony but also raise the risk of getting skin cancer later in life. Heat cramps, while less harmful, can still be uncomfortable and indicate that the body is under significant stress from the heat, which can escalate to more severe problems if not controlled effectively.

Early Warning Signs to Look For

Recognizing early warning symptoms of heat-related disorders is vital for preventing adverse health effects. Early indicators of dehydration in children include dry mouth, reduced urination, dark yellow urine, and thirst. As dehydration worsens, more severe symptoms like lethargy, dizziness, and irritability may appear. For heat exhaustion, early indicators include profuse perspiration, paleness, muscle cramps, and weariness. Children may also feel weak, dizzy, or faint, and could experience nausea or headaches. Parents and caregivers should also be on the watch for signs of disorientation or difficulty concentrating, as these can indicate that the body is struggling to cope with the heat. With sunburn, early warning symptoms include redness and warmth of the skin, which can progress into discomfort and blistering if exposure persists. If these signs are recognized, it is vital to take quick steps to cool the child down, hydrate them, and give adequate skin care to prevent further harm.

Differences Between Heat Exhaustion and Heatstroke

Heat exhaustion and heatstroke are both serious diseases, yet they differ greatly in severity and the immediacy of the threat they pose. Heat exhaustion is often the result of extended exposure to high temperatures, especially when accompanied by physical activity. Symptoms of heat exhaustion consist of profuse perspiration, weakness, disorientation, nausea, and muscle cramps. The skin may feel chilly and damp, and the pulse may be quick and weak. Heat exhaustion can often be treated efficiently by relocating the child to a cooler area, promoting relaxation, and offering water. Nevertheless, if left untreated, heat exhaustion can escalate to heatstroke.

Heatstroke is a medical emergency that happens when the body's temperature regulating mechanism fails, leading to a fast increase in core body temperature, often surpassing 104°F. Unlike heat exhaustion, when sweating is still present, heatstroke often results in heated, dry skin due to the cessation of perspiration. Other symptoms include confusion, convulsions, and loss of consciousness. Heatstroke requires rapid medical attention, as it can lead to severe organ damage or death. The major difference between the two conditions rests in the body's ability to regulate temperature; in heat exhaustion, the body is still working to cool itself, whereas, in heatstroke, this system has broken down completely, leading to a catastrophic and potentially deadly rise in body temperature.

Long-Term Effects of Heat Exposure

The long-term effects of repeated or severe heat exposure on youngsters can be considerable. Chronic dehydration lead to continuing health complications, including kidney stones and urinary tract infections. Recurrent heat exhaustion may result in permanent weariness and a diminished ability to endure heat in the future. For youngsters who have suffered from heatstroke, the risk for long-term damage is high. Heatstroke can cause irreversible brain damage, leading to cognitive deficits, memory loss, and difficulties concentrating. It can also result in chronic renal damage, cardiovascular difficulties, and a diminished ability to control body temperature, making the individual more susceptible to heat-related disorders in the future.

Additionally, frequent or severe sunburns throughout youth can raise the risk of developing skin cancer later in life. The damage caused by UV exposure accumulates over time, and the more sunburn a youngster receives, the higher their risk of getting melanoma, the worst type of skin cancer. The psychological impact of severe heat-related disorders should not be disregarded either. Children who have had a major heat-related ailment may develop anxiety about heat or outside activities, which can influence their quality of life and willingness to participate in normal childhood activities. Understanding and mitigating these potential long-term impacts is critical for the ongoing health and well-being of children who have been exposed to severe heat.

In addition to the physical health effects, the psychological effects of heat-related disorders on children can be considerable and long-lasting.

Experiencing a severe heat-related condition, such as heatstroke or severe sunburn, can lead to worry or fear of such situations in the future. Children may become extremely cautious about partaking in outside activities, which might hinder their social relationships and physical development. This fear can extend to circumstances that entail heat or sun exposure, even in controlled environments like school playgrounds or summer camps. Over time, this could lead to a reluctance to participate in routine childhood experiences, hurting their overall quality of life.

Moreover, the experience of heat-related illness can create a strain on the family as a whole. Parents and caregivers may acquire heightened anxiety about their child's safety in hot weather, leading to overprotectiveness or excessive worry. This can disrupt family dynamics and create further stress on parents, who may already feel overwhelmed by the responsibilities of keeping their children safe during harsh weather conditions. Educating families about heat-related illnesses and offering them practical measures to prevent these conditions might help alleviate some of these worries, allowing children to enjoy outdoor activities safely.

Another long-term effect of heat exposure in children is the possible impact on academic achievement. Heat stress can affect cognitive skills, as concentration, memory, and decision-making. If a child experiences heat exhaustion or heatstroke, even temporarily, it could damage their ability to function well in school, particularly during warmer months. This can have a cumulative effect on their schooling, leading to gaps in learning and academic progress. In severe situations, the cognitive impairments induced by heatstroke might result in long-term learning issues or developmental delays.

It is necessary to address the broader consequences of climate change on children's health. As global temperatures continue to rise, the frequency and intensity of heatwaves are predicted to increase. This indicates that children today are likely to experience more frequent and severe heat-related dangers throughout their lives. Preparing youngsters to comprehend and manage these hazards is vital not only for their immediate safety but also for their capacity to navigate an increasingly hotter world. By training children and their caregivers with knowledge and resources, we may help prevent the long-term health implications of heat exposure and ensure that they are better prepared to tackle the challenges of a changing environment.

Potential Lasting Health Impacts

Heat-related diseases can have substantial, lasting repercussions on a child's health, particularly if they encounter severe or repeated bouts. Heatstroke, the most deadly of these disorders, can cause lasting damage to the brain and other essential organs. This damage may manifest as cognitive deficits, such as memory loss, trouble concentrating, and impaired mental agility. These neurological changes can have a tremendous impact on a child's capacity to learn and function in school, potentially leading to long-term educational issues.

In addition to cognitive difficulties, severe heat exposure can also affect the cardiovascular system. Children who experience heatstroke may be at a higher risk of developing heart problems later in life. The kidneys, which are vital for filtering waste from the blood and regulating fluid balance, can also suffer long-term harm from dehydration and heat stress. Recurrent dehydration, if not effectively managed, can develop into chronic kidney disease, a condition that can have lifetime repercussions.

Frequent or severe sunburns during childhood also carry significant dangers. The cumulative effect of UV exposure to the skin raises the likelihood of developing skin malignancies, including melanoma, which is one of the most severe kinds of cancer. Early and repetitive sun exposure without sufficient protection can contribute to accelerated aging of the skin, including wrinkles and sunspots, and can also damage the immune system's ability to fight off infections.

The Importance of Early Intervention

Early intervention is crucial in preventing the severe and enduring effects of heat-related diseases in youngsters. Recognizing the early signs of dehydration, heat exhaustion, or sunburn allows parents and caregivers to take quick action to prevent the situation from developing. This can involve relocating the child to a cooler setting, encouraging hydration, applying sunscreen, or seeking medical attention. Prompt treatment not only alleviates immediate discomfort but also minimizes the chance of long-term health concerns.

For diseases like heatstroke, where every minute counts, early action might be the difference between life and death. Rapid cooling of the body and emergency medical treatment are important to prevent the substantial organ damage that can result if the body's temperature remains raised for too long. Educating parents, caregivers, and educators about the significance of early intervention can help ensure that children receive the treatment they need before their condition becomes urgent.

Statistics and Real-Life Stories to Emphasize the Seriousness

Statistics and real-life tales emphasize the seriousness of heat-related illnesses in children and underline the need for attention and early intervention. According to the Centers for Disease Control and Prevention (CDC), heat-related mortality in the United States is highest among children under the age of four. Children account for a major percentage of the almost 700 heat-related deaths that occur in the U.S. each year. Many of these tragedies are preventable with adequate measures and awareness.

A terrible illustration of the dangers of heat-related illnesses happened in 2018 when a one-year-old kid in Phoenix, Arizona, died after being left in a hot automobile. The temperature inside the automobile quickly reached hazardous levels, and despite rescue efforts, the youngster did not survive. This terrible occurrence serves as a clear reminder of how rapidly heat can become lethal for young children, particularly when they are left in surroundings where temperatures can climb within minutes.

Another case from Texas in 2020 included a 10-year-old girl who suffered from heatstroke after a summer soccer practice. Despite the coaches' best efforts, the girl was not immediately recognized as suffering from heatstroke and was not cooled down quickly enough. She survived, but with substantial neurological damage that has impacted her cognitive ability and physical functions. This story underlines the necessity of education and training for people who care for children, particularly in outdoor settings.

These anecdotes and data underline the need for heightened awareness and aggressive steps to safeguard children from the hazards of excessive heat. They also underscore the vital role that early intervention plays in preventing the terrible outcomes that can follow from heat-related diseases.

The experiences of children impacted by heat-related ailments are not just isolated cases; they indicate a bigger public health issue that deserves action. Across the United States, hundreds of children are treated in emergency rooms each year for heat-related illnesses, many of which might have been prevented with basic knowledge and quick management. According to the American Academy of Pediatrics, children are particularly sensitive to heat stress because their bodies are less efficient at regulating temperature, and they are more likely to become dehydrated rapidly.

One troubling piece of data from the CDC shows that from 1998 to 2023, more than 900 children in the U.S. perished from heatstroke after being left in hot cars. These heartbreaking deaths underscore a critical mistake that can occur in even the most well-meaning parents and caregivers. The temperatures inside a vehicle may climb swiftly, even on relatively moderate days, converting a car into a deadly environment in a matter of minutes. Public health campaigns have been established to raise awareness about the dangers of leaving children alone in vehicles, emphasizing the necessity for vigilant care.

In addition to these needless deaths, the long-term effects of heat exposure on children who survive such occurrences can be severe. Children who suffer from severe heatstroke may face years of rehabilitation to restore lost physical and cognitive functions. The psychological trauma of such an encounter can potentially have enduring repercussions, leading to anxiety, sadness, or post-traumatic stress disorder (PTSD).

The significance of early intervention cannot be overemphasized. In instances where children are in danger of heat-related illnesses, prompt and decisive care can prevent the course of symptoms and lessen the chance of long-term damage. This is particularly true for situations like heatstroke, where the window for effective therapy is typically very limited. The importance of recognizing early warning signs—such as excessive perspiration, lethargy, dizziness, or confusion—cannot be emphasized enough. Parents, caregivers, and anyone responsible for children's safety must be armed with the knowledge and means to act immediately when these symptoms are present.

Moreover, it is vital to recognize that while public awareness campaigns and educational measures have helped lower the frequency of heat-related incidents, much work remains to be done. Stories like those of the youngsters in Phoenix and Texas serve as stark reminders of the stakes involved. They also stress the significance of continuing activism and education to ensure that every parent, caregiver, and educator understands the substantial hazards posed by heat exposure and the life-saving importance of early action.

As climate change continues to increase the frequency and intensity of heat waves, these hazards are only going to worsen. This makes it more necessary than ever to take preventive precautions to safeguard children from the dangers of excessive heat. By learning from past catastrophes and providing ourselves with the information to prevent future ones, we can move towards a safer and healthier environment for all children.

Chapter 2

Recognizing Vulnerable Populations

In this situation of heat-related illnesses, it is important to identify and understand the populations most sensitive to severe temperatures. While all children are in danger during heatwaves, specific groups are particularly susceptible to the detrimental effects of high temperatures. These vulnerable populations include newborns and toddlers, children with chronic health issues, and those who may be socially or economically disadvantaged. Recognizing these at-risk populations enables more focused interventions and ensures that the most vulnerable receive the protection they need during periods of excessive heat.

Children at Higher Risk

Children are often more prone to heat-related illnesses than adults due to their smaller body size, faster metabolic rates, and developing physiological systems. They are less efficient at controlling their body temperature and are more to be expected to become dehydrated rapidly. However, within the broad category of children, other groups are at an even higher risk.

Infants and toddlers, because of their age and dependence on caregivers for temperature regulation, are particularly in danger. Additionally, children with chronic health issues, such as asthma, diabetes, or obesity, may have underlying vulnerabilities that make it difficult for their bodies to manage with severe heat.

Infants and Toddlers

Infants and toddlers are among the most vulnerable categories when it comes to heat-related disorders. Their bodies are still developing, and they are unable to control their temperature as effectively as older children or adults. Infants, actually have a greater body surface area relative to their weight, which means they can gain or lose heat more rapidly. This renders them particularly susceptible to both overheating and dehydration, especially in hot conditions. Furthermore, infants and toddlers rely totally on their caretakers to ensure they are kept cool, hydrated, and sheltered from the sun. This dependence increases their risk, particularly if caregivers are not completely aware of the dangers posed by heat or are unable to offer essential care during hot weather.

For example, newborns left in hot cars, even for a short duration, might experience a rapid and deadly rise in body temperature, leading to heatstroke. Toddlers, who may be more mobile but yet cannot understand or articulate their distress effectively, are also in great danger. They may continue to play outside without noticing they are growing warmer, or they may not ask for water when they are thirsty, leaving them more prone to dehydration. These factors add to the heightened risk that excessive heat poses to this age group.

Children with Chronic Health Conditions

Children with chronic health concerns are another category at heightened risk during periods of high heat. Conditions such as asthma, diabetes, heart disease, and obesity can alter how a child's body responds to heat. For instance, children with asthma may find it more difficult to breathe in hot, humid circumstances, which can increase their symptoms and lead to respiratory distress. Diabetes can affect the body's capacity to control fluid balance and glucose levels during heatwaves, raising the risk of dehydration and other problems.

Obesity is another problem that might make it tougher for youngsters to cope with heat. Excess body weight can increase the body's core temperature, making it more difficult to stay cool. Children with obesity may also have poorer tolerance for physical exercise, which might impair their capacity to seek cooler locations or stay hydrated through physical exertion. Additionally, several medications used to treat chronic disorders might impact the body's capacity to regulate temperature or retain fluids, further raising the risk of heat-related illnesses.

Children with chronic health disorders may also experience additional obstacles due to the requirement for continuing medical care, which can be hampered during heat waves. For example, power outages or transportation issues caused by harsh weather can make it tougher for these children to obtain the care they need. This underlines the necessity of having a plan in place to manage chronic diseases during periods of extreme heat and ensuring that caregivers are aware of the unique hazards that heat poses to these vulnerable children.

Overweight and Obese Children

Overweight and obese children are particularly vulnerable to the effects of high heat. surplus body fat functions as insulation, trapping heat in the body and making it harder to discharge surplus temperature. This diminished ability to cool down can lead to a greater core body temperature, even in moderate heat. Additionally, overweight and obese children may have lower levels of physical fitness, which might limit their capacity to engage in activities that assist in controlling body temperature, such as moving to a cooler zone or remaining hydrated through drinking water.

The combination of these variables makes overweight and obese youngsters more prone to heat-related disorders such as heat exhaustion and heatstroke. Physical exercise, even at low to moderate levels, can raise their risk, as their bodies generate more heat and struggle to cool down properly. This is especially concerning for outdoor activities in the summer, where the danger of overheating is already heightened. Caregivers and educators need to be aware of these hazards and take extra precautions to ensure these children remain cool and hydrated during hot weather.

Children with Special Needs

Children with special needs may encounter additional obstacles when it comes to coping with excessive heat. These children commonly have problems that influence their physical or cognitive abilities, making it harder for them to perceive or convey discomfort, thirst, or the need for cooling. For example, a child with autism may have difficulties expressing when they are too hot, or a child with cerebral palsy may struggle to relocate to a cooler area or remove unnecessary clothing. Additionally, some children with special needs may have underlying health concerns or use drugs that further enhance their sensitivity to heat-related disorders.

Caregivers and educators of children with special needs must be diligent in monitoring these youngsters for indicators of heat stress. This involves ensuring that they stay in cool places, remain well hydrated, and avoid excessive physical exertion during periods of extreme heat. It is also crucial to have specific plans in place for managing the unique requirements of these children during hot weather, including tactics for communication and adaptive cooling systems.

Socioeconomic and Environmental Factors

Socioeconomic and environmental factors play a key role in determining a child's risk of heat-related diseases. Children from low-income households may be more likely to reside in dwellings without proper air conditioning or ventilation, increasing their exposure to high interior temperatures. These households may also lack access to resources such as clean drinking water, healthy food, or medical treatment, all of which are crucial for preventing and managing heat-related illnesses. Additionally, children in low-income neighborhoods may have limited access to green spaces or shaded areas where they can play safely outside, further increasing their risk.

Environmental factors, such as urban heat islands, can potentially worsen the effects of heat on children. Urban areas with vast volumes of concrete and asphalt tend to absorb and retain heat, leading to greater temperatures than adjacent rural areas. Children living in these situations are exposed to greater ambient temperatures, increasing their risk of heat-related disorders. Moreover, poor air quality, commonly found in densely populated urban areas, can compound the effects of heat, particularly for children with respiratory disorders.

Addressing these socioeconomic and environmental issues is critical for protecting vulnerable children during periods of high heat. This includes enhancing access to cooling resources, such as air conditioning and clean water, and developing safe outdoor spaces where children can play without the risk of overheating. It also involves raising awareness among caregivers and community leaders about the specific hazards these factors represent and the need to take proactive actions to mitigate them.

Impact of Living Conditions (e.g., Lack of Air Conditioning)

Living conditions play a key role in determining how well youngsters can cope with excessive heat. In particular, the absence of air conditioning can dramatically raise the risk of heat-related disorders. Air conditioning provides a controlled atmosphere where children may cool down, recuperate from heat exposure, and maintain a safe body temperature. Without it, indoor rooms can become dangerously hot, especially during protracted heatwaves. Homes without sufficient ventilation or cooling methods can trap heat, making the indoor environment as harmful as the outdoors. This condition is particularly troubling for families living in older buildings or high-density homes where insulation and airflow may be poor.

Children in houses without air conditioning are more likely to face lengthy periods of heat exposure, which can lead to dehydration, heat exhaustion, or even heatstroke. This risk is heightened for children who are homebound, such as newborns, toddlers, or those with chronic health concerns, who may not have the ability or chance to seek cooler environments. Additionally, families suffering financial difficulties may struggle to afford the electrical costs involved with running fans or air conditioning units, even if they are accessible, leaving youngsters vulnerable to the impacts of high heat.

In some circumstances, families may attempt to cool their houses by opening windows or using fans, but these methods can be insufficient during periods of high heat. Fans can circulate hot air without really lowering the temperature, while open windows can let in additional heat from the outside. As a result, children living in such conditions may be at constant risk, especially during heatwaves, where temperatures remain high even at night, robbing them of the opportunity to cool down and recover from hours of daylight heat exposure.

Influence of Outdoor Activities and Sports

Outdoor activities and sports are crucial for a child's physical development and overall well-being, but during hot weather, they can become harmful. Physical exertion boosts the body's core temperature, and when combined with high ambient temperatures, it can quickly lead to overheating. Children involved in sports or strenuous outdoor play are at heightened risk for heat-related diseases, particularly if they are not provided regular pauses, enough water, and access to shade or cooling locations. The risk is especially significant during the summer months, when temperatures climb, and the strength of the sun's rays is at its peak.

Organized sports, such as soccer, football, and baseball, generally involve extended periods of exertion, and practices or games may be planned during the warmest sections of the day. Coaches and organizers may not always be fully aware of the consequences of heat exposure or may feel forced to continue activities despite the heat. This can lead to circumstances where children are pushed past acceptable boundaries, increasing their risk of heat exhaustion, dehydration, and even heat stroke. Younger children, in particular, may not understand their boundaries or may feel tempted to continue playing despite feeling warm, thereby compounding the risk.

The influence of outdoor activities extends beyond organized sports. Children are naturally energetic and may spend hours playing outside during the summer, often without realizing the dangers of excessive heat. Without sufficient supervision, they may not take critical precautions such as staying hydrated, applying sunscreen, or taking rests in the shade. This can lead to cumulative heat exposure, where the body's ability to cool down is gradually overwhelmed, leading to heat-related disorders.

To reduce these dangers, it is vital to alter outdoor activities and sports during hot weather. This involves scheduling events during cooler times of the day, ensuring children have access to plenty of water, encouraging regular breaks, and constructing shaded rest spots. Educating children, parents, and coaches on the indicators of heat-related illnesses and the significance of water and cooling techniques is also vital. By implementing these actions, the enjoyment and advantages of outdoor activities can be matched with the need to preserve children's health during excessive heat.

Chapter 3

Preventative Measures

Preventative steps are necessary to protect youngsters from the detrimental effects of severe heat. These precautions begin with knowledge and planning, ensuring that both children and their caregivers understand the risks and know how to respond appropriately. Prevention focuses on reducing exposure to heat, ensuring enough hydration, and recognizing early indicators of heat-related illnesses before they escalate. Parents and caregivers should be proactive in monitoring the weather, organizing activities during cooler times of the day, and promoting regular water breaks. Wearing light-colored, loose-fitting clothing can assist reduce heat absorption, while wide-brimmed hats or sunglasses provide further protection from the sun.

Hydration is a vital part of prevention. Children should be told to drink water regularly, even if they do not feel thirsty. It's vital to avoid sugary or caffeinated beverages, which can lead to dehydration. Additionally, caregivers should be diligent about keeping children out of the sun during peak hours, often between 10 a.m. and 4 p.m., when the sun's rays are the greatest. For outdoor activities, ensuring access to shaded places and taking frequent breaks can considerably lower the incidence of heat-related illnesses. Prevention also includes educating children about the significance of being cool and hydrated and empowering them to take care of themselves in hot settings.

Creating a Cool Environment

Creating a cool environment is crucial for protecting children during instances of excessive heat. This covers both indoor and outdoor efforts to decrease heat exposure and keep youngsters comfortable. Indoors, the focus should be on maintaining a temperature that is safe and favorable for rest and healing. This can be performed by utilizing air conditioning, fans, and other cooling methods to lower the temperature and enhance air circulation. It's also crucial to decrease sources of internal heat within the home, such as turning off lights and appliances that generate warmth and closing curtains or blinds to block out direct sunlight.

Outdoors, creating a cool atmosphere requires providing shaded play areas and ensuring that children have access to cooling supplies such as water misters or splash pads. Care should be taken to organize outdoor activities during the cooler periods of the day and to allow adequate opportunity for rest and hydration. On exceptionally hot days, it may be important to limit outside activities altogether and encourage youngsters to play indoors where it is cooler. By promoting a cool environment, both indoors and out, caregivers can greatly lessen the hazards associated with high heat.

Tips for Maintaining a Cool Home Environment

Maintaining a cool home environment involves a combination of measures to keep the indoor temperature at a safe level. One successful option is to use shades, curtains, or blinds to block out the sun's rays during the warmest times of the day. Keeping windows and doors closed during these hours can prevent hot air from entering the home. At night, when the temperature drops, it's advantageous to open windows and allow cooler air to circulate, but this should be done with safety in mind, ensuring that windows are secure and inaccessible to young children.

Fans can assist in circulating air, but they should be used strategically. Placing a fan in front of an open window can help draw cooler air into the room, while ceiling fans can generate a wind-chill effect that makes the area feel cooler. For homes without air conditioning, it's crucial to discover the coolest portions of the house, such as basements or rooms with fewer windows, and use these spaces as a getaway during the hottest hours of the day. It's also suggested to avoid using heat-generating appliances like ovens or stoves during peak heat hours, as these can raise indoor temperatures. Simple modifications, like as switching to energy-efficient lighting or shutting off electronics when not in use, can also help keep the home cooler.

The Role of Air Conditioning and Alternatives

Air conditioning serves a key function in keeping a safe atmosphere during extreme heat. It delivers continuous cooling and can considerably minimize the incidence of heat-related illnesses by keeping indoor temperatures at a safe range. In houses with air conditioning, it's crucial to ensure that the system is running correctly and that filters are clean to maximum efficiency. Regular maintenance of air conditioning devices helps prevent breakdowns during heatwaves when they are most required.

For households without access to air conditioning, alternatives must be sought after to keep the home cool. Fans, while less effective than air conditioning, can nonetheless provide relief by circulating air and providing a cooling effect when utilized properly. Evaporative coolers, commonly known as swamp coolers, are another solution that can be successful in arid conditions. These devices cool the air by evaporating water, which can lower the temperature in a space.

In extreme circumstances, where home cooling choices are insufficient, it may be required to seek out public cooling centers or other air-conditioned locations, such as shopping malls, libraries, or community centers. Spending a few hours in a cooler location can help lower body temperature and lessen the risk of heat-related disorders. Caregivers must plan and know where these resources are located, especially during prolonged periods of excessive heat.

Creating Safe Outdoor Spaces (e.g., Shaded Areas, Water Play)

Creating safe outdoor areas is vital for protecting children from the dangers of severe heat while allowing them to enjoy outside activities. Shaded spaces provide crucial protection from direct sunlight, minimizing the danger of sunburn and overheating. Installing or exploiting natural shade from trees, or building up umbrellas, tents, or canopies, can create cooler spaces where children can play without being exposed to the full intensity of the sun. These shaded locations should be widely accessible and integrated into regions where youngsters are expected to spend most of their time outdoors.

In addition to shade, adding water play into outdoor surroundings is a great way to keep youngsters cool. Water activities, such as sprinklers, splash pads, or even small kiddie pools, provide a fun and engaging method for children to cool down while staying active. Water play helps lower body temperature and minimizes overheating by stimulating regular engagement with water, which evaporates and cools the skin. However, it's crucial to ensure that water play spaces are supervised and safe, with non-slip surfaces and clean, properly kept water to prevent accidents and health concerns.

Hydration Strategies

Hydration is a critical technique for reducing heat-related diseases in children. Ensuring that children drink enough water throughout the day is vital, especially during hot weather. It's crucial to encourage children to drink water often, even before they feel thirsty, as thirst is not usually an early indicator of dehydration. Water should be conveniently accessible, and children should be reminded to take frequent sips, especially during outdoor activities or periods of intense physical effort.

One successful hydration method is to make water more palatable to youngsters by adding slices of fruit like lemon, lime, or berries, which can increase the flavor without adding sugar. Parents and caregivers should also schedule frequent hydration breaks during playtime or sports activities, ensuring that children stop and drink water at defined intervals. For younger children who may not realize the need to hydrate, offering water regularly and modeling healthy hydration practices can help emphasize the significance of being hydrated. Additionally, delivering water-rich foods like watermelon, cucumber, and oranges can aid in overall hydration while offering a refreshing delight.

Importance of Regular Hydration

Regular hydration is vital for sustaining a child's health and well-being, especially in hot weather. Water is necessary for controlling body temperature, supporting metabolic activities, and preserving general health. In the heat, children lose water through sweat, and if this lost fluid is not supplied, it can lead to dehydration. Dehydration can limit a child's capacity to cool down, leaving them more susceptible to heat exhaustion or heatstroke. Ensuring that youngsters are continuously hydrated helps their bodies efficiently handle heat and decreases the danger of overheating.

Children are more prone to dehydration than adults due to their lower body size and faster metabolic rate. This makes regular hydration even more vital for them. Without proper water intake, children may experience weariness, irritability, and difficulty concentrating, which can influence their ability to enjoy and engage in activities. In extreme circumstances, severe dehydration can lead to hazardous health complications that require rapid medical intervention. By prioritizing regular hydration, parents and caregivers can help safeguard children's health during hot weather.

Signs of Dehydration

Recognizing the indications of dehydration in children is crucial for preventing major heat-related disorders. Early indicators of dehydration include increased thirst, dry mouth, and dark yellow urine. As dehydration worsens, children may feel tired, angry, or dizzy. They could also complain of headaches or muscle spasms. It's crucial to note that younger children and newborns may not be able to convey these symptoms properly, so caregivers should be careful in evaluating their behavior and physical health.

More severe indicators of dehydration include dry, chilly skin, fast heartbeat, and quick breathing. In extreme circumstances, dehydration can cause confusion, fainting, and a lack of urination for several hours. If these symptoms arise, it is vital to seek medical assistance quickly, as they suggest that the body is struggling to operate without appropriate fluids. Early action, such as administering water or oral rehydration treatments, can help reverse dehydration and prevent it from progressing into a more serious state. Understanding and identifying these signals early can make a major difference in a child's capacity to recover from heat exposure.

Healthy Drink Options and Hydration Schedules

Choosing healthy drink alternatives and setting a hydration regimen are crucial components of maintaining optimal hydration for children. Water should be the primary beverage for staying hydrated, as it is free of calories, sweets, and chemicals. It effectively restores fluids lost through sweat and helps regulate body temperature. Offering water often throughout the day ensures that youngsters maintain adequate hydration levels.

For variety, parents and caregivers can serve liquids like unsweetened herbal teas or water flavored with fresh fruits and vegetables. Infused water has a pleasant flavor without the additional sugars found in many commercial beverages, making it a better choice for encouraging children to drink more. However, it's vital to avoid sugary drinks such as sodas, fruit juices, or sports drinks, which might contribute to dehydration, rather than avoiding it.

Establishing a hydration regimen helps ensure that youngsters drink enough fluids consistently. For instance, children should drink a glass of water with each meal and at regular intervals throughout the day, particularly before, during, and after vigorous activities. Setting reminders or utilizing a water-tracking app might be good for older children and teens to keep track of their intake. Hydration should be integrated into everyday routines to build a habit of regular fluid consumption.

Age-Appropriate Water Intake Guidelines

Age-appropriate water intake guidelines are necessary for satisfying the hydration demands of children at various stages of development. Younger children, such as toddlers and preschoolers, often require less water than older children but still need to stay well-hydrated. For children aged 1 to 3 years, the general recommendation is roughly 4 cups (about 1 liter) of water per day. Preschoolers aged 4 to 8 years should aim for around 5 cups (nearly 1.2 liters) of water every day.

As children grow, their water needs increase. School-aged youngsters, from 9 to 13 years old, should drink roughly 7 to 8 cups (about 1.6 to 1.9 liters) of water per day. Adolescents aged 14 to 18 require around 8 to 11 cups (approximately 1.9 to 2.6 liters) of water daily, depending on their degree of physical activity and environmental conditions.

These parameters are flexible and should be altered based on factors such as physical activity, temperature, and individual health needs. Monitoring the color of urine—aiming for light yellow—and ensuring that youngsters drink water regularly throughout the day can assist in maintaining optimal hydration levels.

Creative Ways to Encourage Kids to Drink More Water

Encouraging children to drink more water can be tough, but some inventive techniques might make hydration more enticing. One excellent way is to use bright and colorful water bottles or mugs with their favorite characters or motifs. Personalizing their water jugs can make drinking water more pleasurable and interesting for children.

Including water into meals and snacks can also help enhance fluid intake. For example, presenting water-rich fruits like watermelon, cucumber, and oranges, or offering homemade popsicles prepared with fruit juice or pureed fruit, can deliver additional hydration in a delightful form. Another alternative is to prepare water-based smoothies with a variety of fruits and vegetables, which may be both nutritional and hydrating.

Creating a hydration challenge or game might drive youngsters to drink more water. For instance, setting up a daily or weekly goal for water intake and rewarding children for hitting their targets with a small treat or extra playtime will help them stay on track. Additionally, involving children in producing infused water or choosing their favorite fruits for water flavoring can give them a sense of ownership and make the process more pleasurable.

Proper Clothing and Sunscreen Use

Wearing suitable clothing and using sunscreen are crucial steps to protect children from the sun and heat. Clothing should be lightweight, loose-fitting, and constructed from breathable fabrics such as cotton or moisture-wicking textiles. Light-colored clothing is preferable, as it reflects rather than absorbs heat. Avoiding dark or tight-fitting clothes helps lower the danger of overheating and allows for improved airflow, which benefits in cooling the body.

Sunscreen is vital for protecting children's skin from harmful ultraviolet (UV) radiation that can cause sunburn and raise the risk of skin cancer later in life. Broad-spectrum sunscreens with an SPF of 30 or higher should be applied generously to all exposed skin. It's vital to apply sunscreen about 15 to 30 minutes before going outside and to reapply it every two hours, or more frequently if swimming or sweating. Using sunscreen that is water-resistant and developed for children can guarantee that it remains effective during outdoor activities.

Hats with wide brims and sunglasses with UV protection further protect vulnerable areas such as the face, neck, and eyes from the sun's rays. Encouraging children to wear these protective accessories can help insulate them from overexposure and lower the risk of heat-related skin disorders. By combining correct clothes, sunscreen, and protective accessories, caregivers can successfully limit the risk of UV damage and offer a safer outdoor experience for children.

Choosing the Right Fabrics and Styles

Selecting suitable fabrics and clothing patterns is vital for protecting children from heat and sun exposure. Fabrics play a crucial role in how well clothing handles heat and moisture. Opt for lightweight, breathable materials like cotton, linen, or moisture-wicking textiles that allow air to circulate and perspiration to evaporate. These materials help keep the body cooler by facilitating improved airflow and minimizing the danger of overheating.

When choosing clothing styles, select outfits that are loose-fitting rather than tight. Loose clothing allows air to flow easily around the body, which aids in cooling. Additionally, light-colored textiles are desirable since they reflect rather than absorb sunlight, which can help keep the body cooler. Dark-colored clothing absorbs more heat, thereby raising the danger of overheating.

For outdoor activities, select apparel with built-in UV protection. Some fabrics are coated with specific coatings that block damaging UV rays, offering an extra layer of protection against sun exposure. This style of clothing is especially good for longer outdoor activities or children with sensitive skin.

Importance of Sunscreen and How to Use It Effectively

Sunscreen is crucial for protecting children's skin from the harmful effects of ultraviolet (UV) radiation. UV radiation can cause sunburn, and premature skin aging, and increase the risk of skin cancer over time. To provide optimal protection, use a broad-spectrum sunscreen with an SPF of 30 or greater. Broad-spectrum sunscreens save against both UVA and UVB rays, delivering more thorough coverage.

Apply sunscreen generously to all exposed skin, roughly 15 to 30 minutes before going outside. This permission the sunscreen to develop a protecting layer on the skin. Reapply sunscreen every two hours, or more frequently if the youngster is swimming, sweating, or towel-drying. Even water-resistant sunscreens need to be reapplied after water exposure to preserve their effectiveness.

Ensure that the sunscreen is suited for children's delicate skin, which may need to use formulas specifically made for them. Hypoallergenic and fragrance-free sunscreens can lessen the risk of skin discomfort. It's also vital to wear enough sunscreen—about one ounce (a shot glass full) is normally suggested to cover the entire body. For optimal coverage, don't neglect typically missed places like the ears, the back of the neck, and the tops of the feet.

Additional Protective Gear (e.g., hats Sunglasses)

Additional protective clothing is required to further protect children from sun exposure and heat. Hats with wide brims are particularly helpful for protecting the face, neck, and ears from direct sunlight. A hat with a brim of at least 2.5 inches gives more coverage and minimizes the risk of sunburn in these sensitive areas.

Opt for hats manufactured from breathable materials that also provide UV protection.

Sunglasses with UV protection are another critical accessory for safeguarding children's eyes from the sun's harmful rays. Choose sunglasses that block 100% of UVA and UVB radiation to protect the eyes and surrounding skin from any damage. Sunglasses should fit correctly and cover the eyes fully, without gaps. Ensuring that youngsters wear sunglasses regularly can help prevent long-term eye damage and discomfort caused by intense sunshine.

Combining these protective measures with suitable clothes, sunscreen, and supplementary gear helps develop a holistic strategy for sun and heat protection. By integrating these techniques, caregivers can successfully lower the risk of heat-related health issues and offer a safer and more enjoyable experience for children in hot weather.

Chapter 4

Cooling Strategies at Home

Effective cooling measures at home are vital for maintaining a comfortable and safe environment, especially during seasons of excessive heat. For families without air conditioning, it is crucial to seek alternate strategies to keep indoor spaces cool and lower the risk of heat-related problems.

Explore Options for Families Without Air Conditioning

For families lacking air conditioning, there are various practical techniques to maintain indoor temperatures. One successful way is to utilize fans to circulate air and produce a cooling breeze. Ceiling fans, box fans, and oscillating fans can help move air about a space and provide some relief from the heat. Placing a dish of ice in front of a fan can boost the cooling effect by adding moisture to the air.

Another method is to use cooling towels or ice packs to reduce body temperature. Drape a cooling towel over the neck or apply ice packs to pulse sites like the wrists and ankles to help cool down. Additionally, spending time in the early morning or late evening when temperatures are lower can help avoid the peak heat of the day.

Suggest Alternatives Like Visiting Libraries, shopping malls, or Designated Cooling Centers

When home cooling solutions are insufficient, seek alternative destinations to escape the heat. Public places such as libraries, shopping malls, and community centers often have air conditioning and can provide a cool shelter during the hottest parts of the day. These venues are often open to the public and offer a comfortable place to rest and stay cool.

Designated cooling centers are another resource to consider. Many municipalities set up cooling centers throughout this extreme heat events to offer a safe, air-conditioned environment for people. These centers can be accessed through local government websites, community newsletters, or emergency services. Ensuring that families are aware of these options and how to access them can help them manage heat more efficiently.

Offer Tips for Keeping Indoor Spaces Cooler

Keeping indoor rooms cooler can considerably increase comfort during hot weather. Start by closing shades and drapes during the day to block off direct sunlight, which can elevate indoor temperatures. Using reflective or light-colored window coverings can help reduce heat intake from the sun.

Another option is to open windows during the cooler hours of the morning and evening to allow fresh air to circulate in the home. During the day, keep windows and doors closed to prevent warm air from entering.

Opting for lower floors in a multi-story home can also help, as heat rises and upper floors tend to be hotter. If possible, use the lower floors for sleeping or resting during the warmest hours of the day.

Using appliances that generate heat, such as ovens or stoves, during cooler periods of the day or choosing no-cooked meals can also assist in maintaining a lower indoor temperature. In addition, shutting off lights and electronics while not in use minimizes the amount of heat created indoors.

Implementing these methods can help create a more comfortable living environment and guard against heat-related health risks, especially in houses without air conditioning.

Fan Usage and Limitations

Fans are a crucial tool for cooling indoor environments, particularly in households without air conditioning. They function by producing airflow, which helps drain sweat from the skin and so gives a cooling effect. This can make the surroundings feel colder and more comfortable, especially when the humidity is low. In the absence of air conditioning, fans may effectively circulate air and create a breeze, making it easier to moderate indoor temperatures.

When Fans Are Helpful (Especially if No Air Conditioning Is Available)?

Fans can be particularly useful during mild heat when air conditioning is not accessible. They help promote airflow and provide a wind-chill effect that can make the room feel several degrees cooler. For example, positioning a fan near an open window might draw cooler outside air into the home and push hot indoor air out. This approach, known as cross-ventilation, can considerably reduce indoor temperatures when employed successfully.

In addition, employing fans at night can help cool down the living space as the outside temperature decreases. By situating a fan to blow cold night air into the home, you may benefit from the lower temperatures outside and help lower the internal temperature.

Caution Against Using Fans During Extreme Heat

While fans are useful in many settings, they have limitations, especially during intense temperatures. When temperatures climb dramatically, fans alone may not provide sufficient cooling and can sometimes add to heat-related health hazards. Fans circulate air but do not lower the temperature of the space; therefore, under particularly hot conditions, they may just push around hot air, making it feel warmer rather than cooler.

Using fans during excessive heat without additional cooling methods can lead to an increased risk of heat exhaustion or heat stroke, particularly for vulnerable groups such as children and the elderly. In such settings, it is crucial to combine fan usage with other cooling methods, such as staying hydrated, wearing light clothing, and taking advantage of cooler locations like public spaces with air conditioning.

Address Safety Concerns Related to Fan Placement

Proper placement and use of fans are vital to ensuring safety and efficacy. Place fans on sturdy surfaces and ensure they are positioned away from areas where they can provide a tripping hazard. Avoid positioning fans too close to flammable things, such as drapes or paper, to prevent potential fire hazards.

When using a fan while sleeping, ensure that it is positioned correctly and does not come into contact with bedding or other objects. For ceiling fans, check that they are securely mounted and in good working order to prevent accidents. Regularly clean fans to remove dust and debris, which can not only damage performance but also pose health problems if collected dust is blown throughout the room.

Understanding the right usage and limitations of fans, as well as implementing important safety precautions, families may efficiently manage indoor temperatures and create a safer and more comfortable living environment during hot weather.

Chapter 5

Safe Outdoor Play and Activities

When it is hot outside, it is crucial to take steps to safeguard the safety of children, even if children need to engage in outdoor play and activities since it is beneficial to their physical and mental well-being. Because prolonged exposure to high temperatures can result in heat-related illnesses, parents and caregivers must pay attention to the schedule, length, and conditions of activities that take place outside.

Timing and duration of Outdoor play

Both the timing and the duration of time spent playing outside are important considerations in the prevention of heat-related illnesses. To reduce the likelihood of experiencing heat exhaustion or heat stroke, it is essential to schedule activities that take place outside during the cooler portions of the day. During hot weather, it is recommended that children play for shorter periods, with regular breaks offered in settings that are shaded or air-conditioned. This will allow them to calm down and rehydrate.

Best Time for Outdoor Activities

Early in the morning or late in the evening, when temperatures are lower and the sun's intensity is lower, are often the optimum times for activities that take place outside when the weather is hot. As a result of the fact that the morning hours, which start at 6:00 a.m. and last until 10:00 a.m., are typically the coolest portion of the day, this is the perfect time for youngsters to play outside. As a similar point of reference, after six o'clock in the evening, the sun starts to set, and temperatures begin to decrease, which presents still another opportunity for safer outside play.

During these periods, children can engage in physical activities like jogging, playing sports, or exploring nature without being exposed to the highest levels of heat. It is also advised to seek shaded settings or parks with tree cover to further limit the risk of overheating.

Limiting Exposure During Peak Heat Hours

Limiting exposure during peak heat hours, often between 10:00 a.m. and 4:00 p.m., is vital for safeguarding youngsters from the detrimental effects of the sun and high heat. During these hours, the sun is at its highest point in the sky, and UV radiation is most powerful, increasing the likelihood of sunburn and dehydration.

If outdoor activities must occur during these hours, it is vital to take extra measures, such as giving adequate fluids, using sunscreen with a high SPF, and ensuring children wear protective clothes, hats, and sunglasses. Additionally, play periods should be kept brief, with regular pauses in cool, shady settings to reduce overheating.

By carefully arranging the timing and duration of outside activities, and by making efforts to limit exposure during the hottest periods of the day, parents and caregivers can help ensure that children stay safe and healthy while still enjoying the benefits of outdoor play during the summer months.

Planning Safe Outdoor Activities

Planning safe outdoor activities during hot weather needs careful consideration of the environment, timing, and types of activities to ensure that children may enjoy the outdoors without jeopardizing their health. Choosing activities that help youngsters to stay cool while being active is key. Parents and caregivers should prefer shaded places, water-based activities, and chances for regular breaks. Additionally, it is vital to modify the intensity of activities dependent on the temperature and humidity to avoid overheating.

Incorporating Water Play to Keep Cool

Incorporating water play into outdoor activities is a fantastic approach to help youngsters stay cool while having fun. Water sports, sprinklers, and small pools can provide a much-needed reprieve from the heat and are often more pleasant for children than traditional land-based activities during hot weather. Simple activities like running through a sprinkler, playing with water balloons, or splashing in a kiddie pool may be both relaxing and interesting.

It is necessary to observe youngsters closely during water play to guarantee their safety. Even shallow water can provide a drowning risk, therefore constant adult supervision is essential. Additionally, parents and caregivers should ensure that children are wearing adequate swimwear, sunscreen, and protective gear like water shoes to prevent slips and falls.

Safe Sports Practices During Hot Weather

Sports are a frequent outdoor activity for children, but during hot weather, it is vital to apply safe techniques to prevent heat-related illnesses. Coaches, parents, and caregivers should schedule practices or games during cooler hours of the day, such as early morning or late evening. If activities must take place during warmer hours, they should be adapted to lessen physical intensity, and more frequent water breaks should be mandated.

Children should be encouraged to wear lightweight, breathable clothing and to drink plenty of fluids before, during, and after sporting activities. Coaches should be trained to recognize the early signs of heat exhaustion and heat stroke and to act swiftly if a youngster develops symptoms. Cooling stations with shade, cold water, and fans should be accessible throughout sporting events to help children cool down when needed.

How Parents and Caregivers Can Protect their Children During Outdoor Activities

Education is crucial to ensuring that children are protected during outdoor activities in hot weather. Parents and caregivers should be informed about the risks of heat-related illnesses and the need to take preventive measures. They should recognize the indicators of dehydration, heat exhaustion, and heat stroke, and know how to respond if a kid exhibits these symptoms.

Practical advice for protecting children includes dressing them in proper attire, applying sunscreen periodically, ensuring they drink enough water, and providing access to shaded or air-conditioned spaces. Parents and caregivers should also be aware of the local weather forecast and schedule activities appropriately, avoiding outdoor play during excessive heat advisories.

By educating parents and caregivers with the knowledge and skills to protect children during outdoor activities, we can create a safer environment for children to enjoy the benefits of outdoor play, especially during the warmest months of the year.

Emphasize Lightweight, Breathable Clothing Choices

Choosing the right attire is essential for keeping youngsters comfortable and safe during hot weather. Lightweight, breathable fabrics such as cotton or moisture-wicking materials help to regulate body temperature by allowing air to circulate and perspiration to dissipate. Loose-fitting clothing is also ideal, as it encourages greater airflow and decreases the risk of overheating. Light-colored garments are advised because they reflect, rather than absorb, the sun's rays, keeping the body cooler. Parents should avoid synthetic clothes that can trap heat and moisture, leading to discomfort and an increased risk of heat-related illnesses.

Encourage Frequent Breaks and Shade-Seeking Behavior

In hot weather, children need to take regular breaks to cool down and prevent heat-related diseases. It is crucial to teach youngsters the habit of finding shade often during outside activities. Whether enjoying sports, engaging in water play, or simply running around, children should be encouraged to relax in shady locations to lower their body temperature and avoid excessive sun exposure.

Setting up dedicated rest spaces with shade and access to cool drinks will help promote this behavior. Parents and caregivers should advise children to take breaks every 15 to 20 minutes, especially during intensive activity. These pauses provide an opportunity for children to hydrate, apply sunscreen, and cool off before resuming play.

Educating Children on Heat Safety

Educating children about heat safety is vital in helping them recognize the signs of overheating and understand the need to take precautions. Children should be taught the basic principles of remaining safe in hot weather, such as drinking water regularly, seeking shade, and wearing suitable clothing. Simple explanations targeted to their age level can help them grasp these concepts and make better judgments when playing outside.

In addition, children should be aware of the symptoms of heat-related diseases, like dizziness, nausea, or excessive perspiration, and encouraged to alert an adult promptly if they feel poorly. By providing children with knowledge about heat safety, parents and caregivers can help them become active participants in safeguarding their health during hot weather. This instruction can be reinforced through interesting activities, such as games or role-playing, to make the learning experience engaging and memorable.

Teach Children to Recognize When They're Overheated

Youngsters must learn how to notice when their bodies are becoming hot, as this awareness can prevent major heat-related illnesses. Children should be taught to pay attention to certain signals that indicate they may be overheated. These indicators include feeling dizzy, lightheaded, or unusually weary; getting headaches; feeling extremely sweaty or, conversely, not sweating at all despite being hot; and recognizing that their skin feels clammy or unusually warm to the touch.

Parents and caregivers can use age-appropriate terminology to help youngsters grasp these symptoms. For example, explaining that if they start to feel "funny," "tired out," or "too hot," they need to quit what they're doing and find a cooler spot. Reinforcing the idea that it's alright to take a break and that identifying these indicators is a sign of being clever and taking care of oneself helps encourage children to listen to their bodies and act fast when they need to calm down.

Encouraging Self-Care and Awareness

Encouraging children to practice self-care and develop a feeling of awareness about their bodies is an important component of heat safety. Teaching children that taking care of themselves is a sign of strength, not weakness, helps them feel accountable for their well-being. This includes urging children to drink water regularly, take rests in the shade, and wear sun-protective gear.

Parents and caregivers should urge youngsters to speak up if they start to feel too hot or uncomfortable. Creating an open environment where children feel safe to share how they're feeling without fear of being advised to "tough it out" is vital. Self-care can also be included in daily routines, where children are encouraged to check in with themselves about how they feel throughout their activities.

In addition, integrating youngsters into the decision-making process regarding their safety can further strengthen their awareness. For example, letting children choose between different types of cool drinks or allowing them to pick out their caps or sunglasses can make them more inclined to engage in these protective actions. By promoting a proactive approach to self-care and awareness, children are better equipped to manage their health in hot weather, minimizing the risk of heat-related disorders.

Reinforcing Good Habits Through Positive Reinforcement

Building long-lasting habits around self-care and heat safety is most effective when positive reinforcement is utilized consistently. Praising children when they make good decisions, such as taking a break when they feel overheated or drinking water without being reminded, can encourage these behaviors. Positive reinforcement might include verbal praise, little rewards, or additional privileges, all of which help to encourage the continued practice of these vital practices.

Parents and caregivers can also set up a system where children earn points or stickers for practicing proper heat safety, which can be traded for a special gift or activity. This not only makes the process fun but also helps children grasp the need to stay safe in the heat in a positive, engaging way.

Creating a Supportive Environment

Creating an environment where children feel supported in their efforts to be cool and safe is crucial to ensure they absorb these habits. This includes more than just delivering instructions; it also requires modeling the habits you wish to see in your children. When parents and caregivers consistently practice heat safety—such as by wearing hats, seeking shade, and staying hydrated—they establish a powerful example that children are likely to follow.

It's also crucial to establish clear and consistent guidelines for outside play during hot weather. For instance, designating precise periods for outdoor activities, encouraging regular water breaks, and ensuring that shaded or cool interior places are always available will help children comprehend and adhere to these requirements. Open communication about why these rules is in place, presented in ways children can comprehend, further reinforces their relevance.

Developing a culture of safety and self-care, children learn that looking after their well-being is not only vital but also a normal part of their daily routine. This supportive setting encourages students to acquire confidence in recognizing and responding to their body's signals, which is crucial in preventing heat-related disorders.

Chapter 6

Emergency Preparedness

Being prepared for emergencies, especially during extreme heat events, is vital for the safety of children. Emergency preparedness involves predicting potential dangers and having a clear, proactive plan to address them. This entails understanding what to do if a child begins to exhibit indications of heat-related illnesses, having a strategy in place for addressing heat waves, and being ready for the likelihood of power outages that could worsen dangerous situations. Effective preparedness can prevent a problem from escalating and ensure that children remain safe and healthy during harsh weather.

Developing a Heat Safety Plan

Creating a heat safety plan is a proactive measure that families may take to protect children during hot weather. This plan should include a list of warning signals for heat-related illnesses like heat exhaustion and heatstroke, along with specific steps to take if these symptoms emerge. The plan should also identify cool spots in the house or neighborhood where children can go to escape the heat, such as air-conditioned rooms, shaded outdoor spaces, or public cooling centers.

Parents and caregivers should discuss the heat safety plan with their children, ensuring they understand what to do if they start feeling too hot. The plan should contain advice on staying hydrated, taking breaks from outdoor activities, and recognizing when it's time to seek help. Additionally, it's crucial to have contact information for medical specialists easily available in case symptoms intensify or if quick care is needed.

What You Can Do If A Child Shows Signs of Heat Exhaustion or Heatstroke

If a kid develops signs of heat exhaustion, such as excessive sweating, weakness, dizziness, nausea, or headache, it's crucial to respond fast. Move the youngster to a cooler spot, have them lie down, and administer cool fluids like water or a sports drink to help with rehydration. Loosen or remove any tight clothing and apply cool, damp cloths to the skin or have the youngster take a cool bath. If symptoms persist or worsen, it's vital to seek medical assistance immediately.

Heatstroke is a medical emergency that requires quick action. If a kid develops signs like a very high body temperature (over 103°F), disorientation, slurred speech, fast breathing, or loss of consciousness, call 911 immediately. While waiting for emergency services to come, relocate the child to a cooler area, remove unnecessary clothing, and try to cool the child down by any means available—using cool water, fans, or cool compresses. Do not offer the youngster anything to drink if they are unconscious or not fully alert.

Outline Steps to Take During a Heatwave or Power Outage

During a heatwave, it's crucial to limit outside activity and keep youngsters indoors as much as possible. Use air conditioning if available, or create cross-ventilation by opening windows on different sides of the home. Keep blinds and curtains closed throughout the day to block out the sun's heat, and avoid using equipment that creates heat, such as ovens or stoves.

In the case of a power interruption during a heatwave, families should be prepared with alternatives for staying cool. Battery-powered fans, chilly baths, and frequent water can assist control body temperature. Identify public locations like libraries, malls, or community centers that may be open and have air conditioning, where the family can go to stay cool. It's also crucial to have an emergency kit ready with necessities like bottled water, portable fans, a battery-operated radio, and first-aid supplies.

Having a defined and trained emergency plan ensures that families can respond rapidly and effectively to safeguard children from the dangers of severe heat, especially in tough circumstances.

When to Seek Medical Attention

Recognizing when to seek medical assistance is crucial in preventing heat-related disorders from becoming life-threatening. Immediate medical treatment should be sought if a kid exhibits signs of severe heat exhaustion or heatstroke, such as continuous vomiting, confusion, fainting, or a body temperature that climbs above 103°F. Any indicators of altered awareness, such as confusion or unresponsiveness, are warning flags that demand urgent medical care. Additionally, if a child's symptoms do not improve fast after attempting to cool them down, or if they worsen, it's crucial to seek professional medical treatment immediately soon. Early action can avert difficulties and assure the child's safety.

Creating an Emergency Contact List

An emergency contact list is an important component of any heat safety plan. This list should include the phone numbers of local emergency services, the child's pediatrician, nearby urgent care centers, and trusted family members or neighbors who can aid in an emergency. It's vital to have this list easily accessible, such as on the refrigerator, in a family binder, or kept on every family member's phone. Additionally, mention the addresses of neighboring hospitals or clinics and directions for getting there. For families with children who have chronic health concerns, contact information for any professionals involved in their care should also be supplied. Ensuring that everyone in the household knows where to find and how to use this list can save significant time during a crisis.

Stress the Importance of Seeking Medical Help Promptly

Promptly seeking medical treatment during a heat-related emergency is not only advisable—it can be lifesaving. Postponements in treatment can lead to the rapid advancement of heat-related disorders, raising the risk of serious consequences or even death. Parents and caregivers must recognize that diseases like heatstroke can progress quickly and require immediate medical action. Emphasizing the need to respond immediately, without hesitation, when symptoms first occur will help prevent long-term health implications and provide the best possible outcome for the kid. When in doubt, it is always preferable to err on the side of caution and seek professional medical counsel.

Basic First Aid for Heat-Related Illnesses

Knowing basic first aid for heat-related disorders can make a major difference in an emergency. For heat exhaustion, start by relocating the kid to a cooler setting, preferably indoors or in the shade. Encourage the youngster to drink cool fluids—water or an electrolyte solution is good. Loosen any tight clothing and apply cool, damp towels to the skin, or have the youngster take a cool bath to reduce their body temperature. If the child's health does not improve within 30 minutes, or if they begin to show indications of heatstroke, seek medical assistance immediately.

For heatstroke, quick action is important. Begin by contacting 911 or bringing the youngster to an emergency room as quickly as possible. While waiting for aid to arrive, relocate the youngster to a cooler spot and remove unnecessary clothing. Use any possible means to cool the youngster down—such as immersing them in a chilly bath, sponging them with cool water, or using fans to circulate air around them. Do not offer the youngster anything to drink if they are unconscious or not fully alert. The goal is to lower the body temperature as rapidly as possible while waiting for professional medical intervention.

By being prepared with these first aid techniques and recognizing when to seek medical help, parents and caregivers can effectively respond to heat-related situations, guaranteeing the safety and well-being of their children.

Steps to Take Before Help Arrives

When a youngster is having a heat-related sickness, taking prompt action before expert help arrives is vital. The first action is to take the youngster to a cool, shaded area to prevent future exposure to heat. Remove any superfluous clothing to assist their body cool down more effectively. If the child is conscious and attentive, encourage them to drink cool water or an electrolyte solution to help replace fluids and reduce their body temperature. Applying cool, damp towels to their skin, particularly on the forehead, neck, armpits, and groin, can also help drop their temperature. If feasible, fan the youngster gently or use a spray bottle to sprinkle their skin with cool water. The goal is to stabilize the child's condition and keep it from worsening until medical help comes.

Importance of Quick Action

Acting early in response to indicators of heat-related sickness can be the difference between a mild case and a life-threatening emergency. Heat-related disorders, such as heat exhaustion and heat stroke, can progress rapidly, with potentially fatal effects if not managed swiftly. Every minute counts when dealing with these illnesses, and delaying action can lead to severe complications, including organ damage or death. By detecting the early signs of heat illness and responding swiftly, parents and caregivers can prevent the condition from developing and lower the risk of long-term health implications. Quick action not only helps in treating the child's immediate symptoms but also provides essential time for medical specialists to take over and offer the necessary care.

Community Resources and Support

In addition to personal readiness, community resources, and support networks play a significant role in protecting children from heat-related illnesses. Many cities offer cooling centers, which are secure, air-conditioned areas where families can seek sanctuary during intense heat. Public facilities such as libraries, community centers, and malls can also serve as a short reprieve from the heat. Parents and caregivers must be aware of these resources, especially if their home lacks air conditioning or other effective cooling methods.

Local health departments and community organizations typically provide educational resources on heat safety, including suggestions on reducing heat-related illnesses and information on available community support. These groups may also offer support programs for families in need, such as supplying fans, air conditioning systems, or financial help with utility costs during heatwaves. Engaging with these community services can provide additional layers of protection for children and ensure that families have access to the support they need to keep their children safe during hot weather.

Local Resources for Heat Relief

During seasons of high heat, families must know about local resources available for heat relief. Many municipalities build cooling facilities where citizens can find reprieve from hot heat. These facilities are often set up in public buildings like community centers, libraries, or churches and provide air-conditioned surroundings where families can keep cool and protected. Some communities also give free transportation to these locations for those who may not have a way to get there. In addition to cooling facilities, public parks featuring water features, such as splash pads, can be a terrific method to keep children cool while allowing them to play safely outdoors.

Local health departments and emergency management agencies generally retain up-to-date information about available resources during heatwaves, including locations of cooling facilities, hours of operation, and other services such as water distribution stations. It's crucial to be aware of these resources, especially for families without air conditioning at home. Staying connected with local community groups, and social media, or subscribing to alerts from local authorities will guarantee that you receive timely information about heat relief choices.

How to Access Emergency Services

In the event of a heat-related emergency, understanding how to rapidly reach emergency assistance is crucial. The first step is to phone 911 if a child is experiencing severe symptoms such as confusion, unconsciousness, or if they cease sweating, as these can be signals of heatstroke, a life-threatening condition. When contacting emergency services, provide clear and concise information about the incident, including the child's symptoms, location, and any first aid steps you have already taken.

In some locations, there may also be specific hotlines or services set up during extreme heat events to aid citizens. For example, several cities have specific lines for non-emergency heat-related concerns, where you can get advice or be sent to the nearest cooling center. It's a good idea to familiarize oneself with these local numbers and services before an emergency arises.

For families living in rural areas or places with limited emergency response resources, it is particularly crucial to have a strategy in place for getting emergency services swiftly. This can include identifying the nearest hospital or urgent care facility, ensuring that your vehicle is in good functioning shape, and learning alternate routes in case of road closures or traffic. Being prepared and knowing how to seek emergency services can make a major difference in safeguarding children from the hazards of extreme heat.

Chapter 7

Special Considerations for Schools and Daycares

Schools and daycares are critical in sheltering children from the dangers of severe heat. These surroundings are accountable for the well-being of large groups of children for extended durations, making it vital that they develop and enforce comprehensive heat safety measures. With children spending substantial periods of their day in these settings, parents must understand and ensure that proper steps are being taken to safeguard their children from heat-related dangers.

School Policies and Procedures

To effectively handle heat concerns, schools and daycares must have well-defined rules and procedures in place. These regulations should contain recommendations for monitoring the temperature and determining whether outdoor activities should be changed or canceled. For example, schools should establish rules for transferring outdoor activities indoors when temperatures increase to dangerous levels. Additionally, regulations should cover hydration, requiring regular water breaks, and ensuring children have easy access to drinking water throughout the day. Educators and caregivers should also be trained to recognize the indicators of heat-related diseases and be prepared to take early action if a kid develops symptoms.

Ensuring Schools Have Heat Safety Protocols

Parents should feel empowered to ask schools and daycares about their heat safety practices. Ensuring that these institutions have a clear and effective plan can provide peace of mind and help reduce heat-related catastrophes. Schools should undertake regular assessments and drills of their heat safety protocols, ensuring that all staff members are aware of the processes. In places where high temperatures are regular, schools should consider introducing early dismissal policies on days when the heat index reaches harmful levels. Regular communication with parents on heat safety measures is also vital, keeping them informed and aligned with the school's efforts to protect children.

Importance of Shaded Playgrounds and Indoor Recess Options

The physical environment of schools and daycares is another crucial aspect of protecting children from heat. Playgrounds should be provided with adequate shaded places where children can play without being directly exposed to the sun. Shade can be produced by natural methods, such as trees, or with manmade structures like canopies or shade sails. These spaces should be carefully positioned above play equipment and areas where children are expected to spend the most time.

In addition to covered outdoor places, schools should have inside recess options available when the heat gets too oppressive. Indoor activities can include gymnasium games, creative arts, or quiet time in air-conditioned classrooms. By providing these alternatives, schools can ensure that students stay active and engaged without risking heat exposure.

Educating Caregivers and Staff

Training caregivers and school workers on heat safety is vital for properly managing heat-related dangers. Education should cover the detection of heat-related illnesses, including symptoms of heat exhaustion and heatstroke, and the necessary procedures to take when these symptoms are noticed. Training programs can also include information on prevention measures, such as recognizing signs of dehydration and the necessity of maintaining a cool atmosphere for children. Regular refresher courses and updates on heat safety rules will help ensure that staff stay knowledgeable and prepared to act rapidly in response to heat-related crises.

Training for Recognizing and Responding to Heat-Related Illnesses

Proper training for recognizing and responding to heat-related illnesses is crucial for caregivers and personnel. This training should give extensive information on the signs of heat exhaustion, such as excessive perspiration, weakness, dizziness, and nausea, and heatstroke, characterized by a high body temperature, quick pulse, and confusion. Staff should be educated on quick activities to take, including relocating the kid to a cooler environment, applying cool compresses, and encouraging water. Training should also emphasize the significance of alerting emergency services when a child's health does not improve or worsen. Role-playing scenarios and hands-on experience can help ensure that personnel are confident and skilled in resolving heat-related issues.

Importance of Hydration Breaks and Monitoring

Regular hydration breaks are a crucial aspect of any heat safety strategy. Caregivers and staff should ensure that children have regular opportunities to drink water throughout the day, especially during periods of high heat. Water should be available and easily accessible to all children. Monitoring hydration levels is also crucial; caregivers should be aware of indicators that a child may not be drinking enough water, such as dry mouth, dark urine, or lethargy. Implementing periodic water breaks and encouraging children to drink often, even if they do not feel thirsty, can help reduce dehydration and heat-related diseases.

Communicating with Parents

Effective communication with parents about heat safety is vital for a coordinated strategy to minimize heat dangers. Schools and daycares should provide regular updates on heat safety precautions, including any adjustments to outside activities or schedules due to high temperatures. Informing parents about the procedures taken to protect their children, such as instituting hydration breaks and monitoring for heat-related illnesses, helps create trust and ensures that parents are aligned with the institution's efforts. Additionally, schools and daycares should offer advice to parents on how they can support heat safety at home, including tips on hydration, suitable clothes, and recognizing heat-related symptoms. Keeping open channels of communication allows for a collaborative effort to safeguard children's health during hot weather.

How Schools Can Keep Parents Informed

Schools can keep parents informed about heat safety precautions through numerous effective communication channels. Regular updates can be supplied through school newsletters, emails, and phone calls, describing current heat safety measures and any modifications to school activities due to high temperatures. Schools should also employ their websites and social media networks to disseminate relevant information and reminders about heat safety. In cases of excessive heat, schools can consider sending out immediate alerts to ensure that parents are aware of any urgent modifications to the daily schedule or additional precautions being taken. Hosting instructional sessions or webinars can also help educate parents and provide a forum for addressing heat safety techniques and answering any questions they may have.

Importance of Home-School Coordination in Hot Weather

Coordination between home and school is crucial for efficiently controlling heat risks. When parents and schools work together, they can guarantee that children receive consistent messages and support on heat safety. This relationship is vital for promoting hydration measures, monitoring for symptoms of heat-related illnesses, and making appropriate changes to activities. Schools should explain their heat safety plans to parents, including specifics on how outside play will be supervised and what safeguards are in place for keeping children cool. Conversely, parents should inform schools of any specific considerations for their children, such as medical issues that may enhance heat sensitivity. By maintaining open lines of communication and sharing information, both parties may work to create a safe and supportive environment for children during hot weather.

Traveling with Children

Traveling with children during hot weather demands extra planning to protect their safety and comfort. When traveling, whether by vehicle, bus, or airline, it's necessary to prepare for the potential obstacles provided by hot temperatures. Keep a supply of water accessible and urge youngsters to drink often to stay hydrated. In autos, ensure that the vehicle is well-ventilated and that air conditioning is used effectively. Plan stops on long trips to allow youngsters to rest in cooler environments and to rehydrate. If traveling by public transit, be aware of the availability of air-conditioned spaces and plan accordingly.

When traveling, carefully consider the availability of shade and cooling options at your destination. Pack lightweight, breathable clothing for children and bring along required sun protection, such as sunscreen, hats, and sunglasses. Acquaint yourself with the location of emergency services and cooling centers in the neighborhood. Preparing for potential heat-related difficulties in advance can help provide a safer and more comfortable travel experience for children during hot weather.

Researching Heat Conditions at Destinations

Before going, it is crucial to examine the heat conditions at your location to ensure you are prepared for the climate. Start by reviewing the weather forecast for the duration of your trip to understand the predicted temperatures and heat advisories. Look for information on local climatic patterns, such as common heat waves or periods of high humidity, which can affect your vacation plans. Additionally, seek out any specific health warnings or heat-related alerts issued by local authorities. This information will help you plan appropriate activities and make necessary adjustments to your holiday itinerary. Understanding the heat conditions of your destination allows you to make proactive efforts to ensure your children's health and comfort throughout the trip.

Packing Heat-Safety Essentials

When preparing for a trip during hot weather, add goods that will help manage and limit heat exposure. Essential goods to pack should include:

Hydration Supplies: Bring sufficient water bottles or a portable water filter to ensure access to clean drinking water at all times. Consider incorporating electrolyte tablets or drinks to help restore critical minerals lost via sweating.

Cooling Items: Pack cooling towels or portable fans to help keep children comfortable in hot situations. A tiny, battery-operated fan can be particularly useful for travel and outdoor activities.

Sun Protection: Include sunscreen with a high SPF, as well as hats with brims and sunglasses to guard against UV rays. Choose sunscreen that is water-resistant and safe for children's sensitive skin.

Appropriate apparel: Select lightweight, breathable apparel made from moisture-wicking textiles. Long-sleeved shirts and long pants in light colors can offer additional protection from the sun while still being comfortable in hot weather.

First Aid Kit: Ensure your first aid kit has products for treating heat-related illnesses, such as aloe vera gel for sunburn, and bandages for small injuries. Having a thermometer can also help monitor body temperature if heat-related symptoms emerge.

Cooling Packs: Consider bringing gel or ice packs that can be used to chill down if needed. These packs might be particularly helpful if you encounter unexpected heat or if air conditioning is unavailable.

By carrying these essentials, you can better limit heat exposure and help keep your children safe and comfortable throughout your trip.

Chapter 8

The Role of the Community in Protecting Children

The community plays a critical role in safeguarding children from heat-related hazards. By working together, community members may build environments that promote children's well-being during hot weather. This collective endeavor involves multiple stakeholders, including local government agencies, schools, healthcare providers, and community organizations. Each group contributes to developing a support network that promotes the effectiveness of heat safety measures. Community involvement might include arranging cooling centers, encouraging heat safety awareness, and offering services for families in need. Engaging in proactive and collaborative measures helps to guarantee that children remain safe and healthy during periods of excessive heat.

Community Outreach and Education

Community engagement and education are crucial components in the fight against heat-related disorders. Effective outreach entails providing information about heat safety through numerous channels, such as community centers, local events, and social media platforms. Educational programs can be adapted to serve the special requirements of diverse community groups, including parents, caregivers, and educators. Workshops and seminars can offer practical guidance on preventing heat-related illnesses, recognizing signs, and taking necessary responses. Collaboration with local media can further increase the reach of these educational activities, ensuring that essential information reaches as many people as possible. By prioritizing outreach and education, communities may empower individuals with the information and resources needed to safeguard children from heat-related threats.

Public Health Campaigns and Initiatives

Public health campaigns and initiatives are crucial in raising awareness about heat safety and encouraging collective action. These campaigns can be intended to inform the public about the risks of heat exposure and the procedures necessary to mitigate these risks. Initiatives may involve distributing instructional booklets, running advertising on local television and radio, and arranging community activities focused on heat safety. Public health authorities can cooperate with schools, local businesses, and nonprofit organizations to raise public awareness and encourage best practices. Campaigns frequently emphasize on the necessity of water, detecting symptoms of heat-related illnesses, and the availability of community facilities such as cooling centers. By utilizing these programs, communities may develop a culture of prevention and preparedness.

Importance of Educating the Broader Community

Educating the larger community is crucial to managing heat-related issues successfully. Knowledge about heat safety should extend beyond individual households to include all members of the community. When the larger community is aware, it fosters a supportive climate where everyone participates in safeguarding children. Education activities can help debunk myths regarding heat exposure and improve proper understanding of protective actions. Informed community members are better positioned to take preventive action, offer aid to those in need, and lobby for required resources and legislation. By developing a well-informed community, the collective impact on safeguarding children from heat-related dangers is considerably boosted.

Support for Vulnerable Families

Supporting vulnerable families is vital in safeguarding children from the risks associated with excessive heat. Low-income households sometimes have additional obstacles in regulating heat exposure due to restricted access to resources such as air conditioning and suitable housing. To address these issues, it is crucial to provide specialized help that matches the individual requirements of these families. Community organizations, government agencies, and non-profit groups can work together to design programs that give both immediate aid and long-term answers. Such support not only helps families manage the heat more successfully but also guarantees that children are safe and protected during hot weather.

Providing Resources and Assistance to Low-Income Families

Providing resources and help to low-income families is crucial for efficient heat management. Many low-income households may lack access to air conditioning or other cooling technologies, making it difficult to maintain a comfortable indoor environment during heatwaves. To address this, cities might offer financial assistance programs to help families purchase or repair cooling equipment. In addition, giving away free or low-cost fans, cooling blankets, or portable air conditioning devices can dramatically boost a family's capacity to stay cool. Other forms of support include giving hydration products and organizing programs that enable home visits from health professionals to check on vulnerable households during excessive heat. Ensuring that these tools are easily available will help ease some of the challenges faced by low-income families and protect their children from heat-related health risks.

Community Cooling Centers and Other Support Options

Community cooling centers serve a key role in bringing respite to families without adequate cooling at home. These centers are constructed in inaccessible locations, such as libraries, community centers, and schools, where people can seek sanctuary from the heat. During instances of excessive heat, these facilities provide air-conditioned areas where families may stay cool and hydrated. Local governments and organizations should ensure that information about the locations and operation hours of these facilities is widely publicized through community outreach campaigns. Additionally, other support options may include temporary shelters, transportation services to cooling centers, and partnerships with local companies to offer cooling stations. By providing several support alternatives, communities may help lessen the effects of high heat on disadvantaged families and ensure that children are safe and comfortable during hot weather.

Advocating for Policy Changes

Advocating for legislative reforms is vital in providing a safer environment for children during extreme heat occurrences. Effective policy approaches can create systemic improvements that benefit entire communities. Advocacy activities should focus on persuading local, state, and federal government policies to incorporate stringent heat safety rules. This can involve fighting for the development of minimum cooling requirements for dwellings, improving funding for community cooling initiatives, and supporting research into heat resilience. Advocates can engage with lawmakers, participate in public forums, and partner with community organizations to ensure that heat safety becomes a priority in policy development. By driving these reforms, advocates may help develop a framework that promotes long-term protection for children and vulnerable people during periods of excessive heat.

Encouraging Local Governments to Implement Heat Safety Measures

Local governments play a significant role in implementing and enforcing heat safety measures. Encouraging local governments to adopt and maintain heat safety policies takes several steps. First, community members can share facts and case studies that underscore the need for action, highlighting how heat waves harm public health and safety. Proposals can include drafting or updating local heat response plans, putting up heat alarm systems, and ensuring that cooling centers are sufficiently equipped and accessible. Additionally, local governments might be pressed to integrate heat safety into disaster response strategies and public health campaigns. By actively engaging with local officials and highlighting the benefits of heat safety measures, communities may push the deployment of effective solutions that protect children and other vulnerable groups.

Importance of Urban Planning (e.g., Green Spaces, Tree Planting)

Urban planning is a vital component in minimizing the effects of heat and boosting community resilience. Incorporating green spaces and tree planting into urban development plans can considerably minimize heat exposure and improve overall quality of life. Green spaces, such as parks and community gardens, provide shade and cool the surrounding air through evapotranspiration. Trees and vegetation operate as natural air conditioners, absorbing sunlight and lowering the urban heat island effect, which happens when city areas become much warmer than their rural surroundings. Effective urban planning should incorporate measures for increasing green coverage, constructing cool roofs, and incorporating reflective materials in construction. By prioritizing these factors in city design, communities can create more comfortable surroundings that help shield children from the detrimental impacts of heat and promote public health and well-being.

Protecting children during hot weather is a responsibility that goes across families, communities, schools, and government agencies. The vulnerability of youngsters to heat-related illnesses highlight the need for comprehensive efforts to limit hazards and increase safety measures. In considering the numerous dimensions of heat protection, it is obvious that this issue requires a multi-layered strategy that includes the individual needs of children, the environments in which they are living and play, and the resources accessible to them.

As temperatures continue to rise globally, the risks associated with excessive heat become more obvious, particularly for youngsters, who are less able to control their body temperature and more likely to suffer from dehydration, heat exhaustion, and heatstroke. The necessity to safeguard children from these threats is not simply a matter of comfort but of life and death. Therefore, understanding the important lessons from this conversation is vital for anyone concerned with the care and protection of children.

Summarizing Key

The solutions presented throughout this guide emphasize the significance of creating a safe and cool environment for children during hot weather. From choosing the right attire and ensuring proper hydration to identifying the signs of heat-related illnesses and learning when to seek medical treatment, every aspect plays a crucial role in keeping children safe.

One of the most crucial parts is the establishment of a cool environment, whether at home, school, or during travel. This involves the use of air conditioning, fans, and other cooling methods, as well as initiatives to reduce indoor temperatures by closing shades, using lower floors, and visiting cooler public locations like libraries or malls. In the absence of air conditioning, families might explore numerous options, such as patronizing cooling centers or adopting basic yet effective home-cooling strategies.

Hydration is another key component of heat safety. Ensuring that children drink enough water and consume healthful fluids throughout the day can avoid dehydration, which is a primary cause of heat-related disorders. Parents and caregivers should be aware of the recommended water consumption for children of different ages and be creative in encouraging them to drink more, whether through the use of flavored water, interesting water bottles, or regular reminders. Recognizing the indications of dehydration early on, such as dry mouth, weariness, and dark urine, can help prevent more catastrophic disorders like heat exhaustion and heatstroke.

Proper clothes and the usage of sunscreen are also vital in shielding youngsters from the sun's damaging effects. Lightweight, breathable materials that allow for air circulation, along with broad-spectrum sunscreen and other protective gear like hats and sunglasses, can dramatically lower the risk of sunburn and overheating. Educating youngsters about the need for these precautions and encouraging self-awareness will further boost their ability to be safe in the heat.

Outdoor play is an essential component of a child's growth, but during hot weather, it must be done with prudence. Timing outdoor activities to avoid the hottest portions of the day, ensuring that children take frequent rests in the shade, and including water play are all good strategies to keep them cool. Safe sports practices, such as regulating the intensity of exercises and watching children attentively for signs of overheating, are also required to prevent heat-related illnesses.

Emergency planning is another vital part of protecting children in hot weather. Developing a heat safety plan, knowing what to do if a kid shows indications of heat exhaustion or heatstroke, and recognizing the significance of prompt action can save lives. Having an emergency contact list and understanding when to seek medical treatment are critical components of this plan. Basic first aid skills, such as how to cool down an overheated child or what measures to take before help arrives, can make a major difference in an emergency.

The significance of the community in protecting youngsters from high heat cannot be emphasized. Public health campaigns and community outreach programs play a critical role in educating the larger community about heat safety. Local governments can develop regulations that encourage heat safety measures, such as building community cooling centers and providing resources to low-income families. metropolitan planning that includes green spaces, tree planting, and other cooling methods can also assist minimize the effects of heat in metropolitan settings.

Schools and daycares have a responsibility to protect children during hot weather as well. This involves having heat safety practices in place, ensuring that playgrounds are shaded, and providing indoor recess options when necessary. Educating caregivers and staff on recognizing and responding to heat-related illnesses, as well as ensuring that children stay hydrated, are key measures in reducing heat-related catastrophes. Clear communication between schools and parents is also vital in ensuring that children are safe both at school and at home.

Traveling with children during hot weather demands specific measures. Researching heat conditions at locations, bringing heat-safety items like water, sunscreen, and protective gear, and being prepared for emergencies are all vital actions to ensure that children remain safe when traveling.

The Critical Importance of Protecting Children in Hot Weather

The necessity of protecting youngsters during hot weather cannot be emphasized. Children are more prone to heat-related illnesses due to their smaller body size, faster metabolic rate, and less capacity to regulate their body temperature. As global temperatures continue to rise, the frequency and intensity of heat waves are likely to grow, making it more vital than ever to deploy appropriate heat protection measures.

Children's vulnerability to heat is enhanced by several factors, including their age, health status, and environmental conditions. Infants and toddlers are particularly at risk because they rely on adults to govern their surroundings and provide for their needs. Children with chronic health disorders, such as asthma or heart disease, may also be more susceptible to the effects of heat, as their bodies are less able to cope with temperature extremes.

Socioeconomic and environmental factors can further raise the risk for particular children. Families living in poverty may have limited access to air conditioning or other cooling options, making it more difficult to keep children safe during hot weather. In metropolitan areas, the absence of green spaces and the predominance of heat-absorbing materials can generate "heat islands," where temperatures are much higher than in adjacent rural areas. These variables underscore the need for focused measures to protect the most vulnerable children.

Education is a valuable tool in reducing heat-related illnesses. By teaching children about the dangers of heat and encouraging them to recognize the signs of overheating, parents and caregivers can empower them to take action to protect themselves. This teaching should be age-appropriate and should include practical recommendations, such as staying hydrated, seeking shade, and wearing suitable attire.

Hydration is a vital part of heat safety. Children should be encouraged to drink water regularly, even if they don't feel thirsty. Dehydration can arise quickly in hot temperatures, leading to heat exhaustion or heatstroke if not managed soon. Parents and caregivers should be aware of the indications of dehydration and take steps to ensure that children have access to water throughout the day. In addition to water, various nutritious liquids, such as electrolyte solutions or natural fruit juices, can assist in maintaining hydration.

Clothing also plays a crucial role in shielding youngsters from heat. Light-colored, loose-fitting clothing made from breathable fabrics can help keep youngsters cool by enabling air to circulate and perspiration to drain. In addition, protective clothing, such as hats and sunglasses, can shield youngsters from the sun's rays and lower the risk of sunburn and heat-related illnesses.

Sunscreen is another crucial component of heat safety. Applying broad-spectrum sunscreen with an SPF of 30 or higher can protect children's skin from damaging UV rays. Sunscreen should be applied widely and reapplied every two hours, or more often if the youngster is swimming or sweating. Parents and caregivers should also be cognizant of the need to apply sunscreen to often-overlooked regions, such as the ears, back of the neck, and tops of the feet.

Outdoor play is a crucial element for children, but it requires cautious planning during hot weather. Activities should be organized for the cooler portions of the day, such as early morning or late afternoon, and children should be encouraged to take regular pauses in the shade. Incorporating water play, such as sprinklers or wading pools, can help keep youngsters cool while they enjoy outside activities.

Emergency preparedness is vital in protecting children from the risks of heat. Parents and caregivers should prepare a heat safety plan that includes things to take if a child shows signs of heat exhaustion or heatstroke. This plan should include knowing when to seek medical treatment, how to cool down an overheated child, and what to do during a heatwave or power outage. Having an emergency contact list readily available and knowing the location of the local medical facilities can also help ensure a speedy response in an emergency.

The importance of the community in safeguarding children from heat cannot be underestimated. Public health campaigns and community outreach activities can raise awareness of the dangers of heat and provide services to help families stay safe. Local governments can also play a vital role by implementing policies that encourage heat safety, such as constructing cooling centers, offering financial aid for air conditioning, and incorporating green spaces into urban development.

Schools and daycares have a responsibility to safeguard children from heat-related illnesses during hot weather. This involves having heat safety practices in place, ensuring that playgrounds are shaded, and providing indoor recess options when necessary. Educating caregivers and staff on the signs of heat-related illnesses and the necessity of drinking can help prevent emergencies. Communication between schools and parents is also vital in ensuring that children are safe both at school and at home.

Traveling with children during hot weather demands careful planning and preparation. Parents should investigate the heat conditions at their destination and carry heat-safety items, such as drinks, sunscreen, and protective clothes. Being prepared for emergencies and knowing the location of the nearest medical services can help guarantee that children remain safe when traveling.

Encouraging Proactive and Preventive Approaches

Protecting children from heat-related illnesses demands more than just reactive measures; it necessitates a proactive approach that prioritizes prevention and readiness. Taking proactive precautions can dramatically minimize the likelihood of children experiencing heat-related difficulties and ensure that, when high temperatures occur, families and communities are ready to respond effectively. The emphasis on preemptive interventions is vital, given the growing frequency and intensity of heat waves due to climate change.

One of the most effective preventive tactics is education. Educating both children and adults about the hazards of extreme heat, the indicators of heat-related illnesses, and the significance of drinking and wearing suitable clothing is basic to prevention. Knowledge helps individuals make informed decisions that can prevent the onset of heat-related disorders. Schools, community centers, and healthcare practitioners can all play a part in disseminating this information, ensuring that it reaches every family, especially those in high-risk locations.

Proactive hydration is a vital element in preventing heat-related diseases. Encouraging children to drink water often, rather than waiting until they are thirsty, helps maintain optimal hydration levels. This is especially crucial during periods of physical activity, whether in sports, outdoor recreation, or even routine duties like going to and from school. Parents and caregivers should build routines that combine regular water breaks throughout the day, making it a habitual behavior for children. In addition, understanding the indicators of early dehydration, such as dry mouth, lethargy, and diminished urination, enables for quick intervention before the problem progresses.

Choosing suitable clothing is another key protective measure. Parents should select lightweight, loose-fitting clothing made from breathable fibers for their children. Such clothing helps regulate body temperature by allowing sweat to drain more quickly, which in turn cools the body. Light-colored clothing is better as it reflects rather than absorbs sunlight, lowering the danger of overheating. Beyond ordinary attire, it is vital to consider the individual needs of different activities; for example, sportswear designed to wick away perspiration and keep the body cool might be advantageous during vigorous activities.

Sunscreen application is a preventative measure that should not be disregarded. Regularly applying broad-spectrum sunscreen with an SPF of 30 or higher helps protect children's skin from the harmful effects of UV radiation, which are increase during hot weather. Sunscreen should be applied in every two hours and after swimming or sweating. Teaching children to apply sunscreen independently, under supervision, can create lifelong habits that protect them from skin harm and minimize the risk of skin cancer.

The scheduling of outdoor activities is another area where smart preparation might reduce heat-related difficulties. By planning outside play or sports during the cooler portions of the day—early morning or late afternoon—parents and caregivers can minimize children's exposure to peak heat. If activities must take place during hotter seasons, ensuring that children have access to shaded locations and promoting regular pauses are crucial tactics. Incorporating water-based activities, such as playing with sprinklers or swimming, can also help keep youngsters cool while they enjoy the outdoors.

Creating a heat safety strategy is a vital, proactive step for families. This plan should detail what to do in the event of high heat, including identifying cool locations to go, understanding the signs of heat exhaustion and heatstroke, and knowing when to seek medical treatment. Families should also be aware of local options, such as cooling centers, where they can go if their home becomes too hot. Regularly reviewing and practicing the strategy ensures that everyone knows what to do, avoiding panic and confusion during an actual heatwave.

Community involvement is also an important component of proactive heat protection. Local governments and community organizations can help by providing resources such as free or subsidized cooling equipment, instructional materials, and public service announcements about heat safety. Communities can also arrange volunteer programs to check on vulnerable individuals, such as the elderly and those with young children, during periods of excessive heat. This joint approach ensures that no one is left without the support they need to stay safe.

Schools and daycare organizations should adopt preventative measures as well. Establishing and enforcing heat safety regulations, such as mandated hydration breaks, shaded play spaces, and indoor recess during high heat, can greatly lower the incidence of heat-related illnesses in children. Educating personnel about the indicators of heat exhaustion and heatstroke, as well as training them in basic first aid, ensures that they can respond promptly and effectively in an emergency.

Proactive monitoring of weather forecasts and heat advisories is another crucial habit. Parents, caregivers, and educators should be informed about anticipated heat waves or periods of excessive heat, allowing them to adapt plans and take additional measures. This can require rescheduling outdoor events, ensuring that children are clothed correctly, or arranging provisions for air-conditioned vehicles and locations.

Advocating for and participating in urban design efforts that prioritize heat mitigation can have long-term advantages for communities. Supporting projects that create green spaces, grow trees, and lessen the urban heat island effect can make towns and neighborhoods more robust to heat. These efforts not only protect children but also enhance the general quality of life for all citizens.

Final Thoughts on the Importance of Vigilance in Protecting Children from Heat-Related Illnesses

Vigilance is the cornerstone of protecting children from the risks of high heat. Given the special vulnerabilities of children, who are less capable of regulating their body temperature and more prone to dehydration, parents, caregivers, educators, and communities must remain continually aware of the risks and ready to take action.

The requirement for awareness begins with a solid grasp of the risks connected with heat exposure. Heat-related illnesses can rise quickly, making it crucial for adults responsible for children to recognize the early signs and symptoms. Heat exhaustion, marked by excessive sweating, weakness, and dizziness, can swiftly escalate to heatstroke, a life-threatening condition that requires prompt medical intervention. By remaining aware and sensitive to how children are feeling and behaving, parents can intervene before a situation becomes critical.

Vigilance also entails regular monitoring of environmental conditions. During the summer months, when heatwaves are more frequent, it is vital to be informed about weather forecasts and heat advisories. By keeping track of temperature trends and humidity levels, parents and caregivers can make informed judgments about outside activities, clothing choices, and hydration needs. This continual awareness enables the prompt deployment of preventive actions, such as postponing activities or seeking out cooler locations.

In the context of daily routines, vigilance implies forming and sustaining behaviors that prioritize heat safety. This involves ensuring that children drink water regularly, wear suitable clothing, and apply sunscreen before going outside. It also requires creating guidelines for outdoor play, such as taking pauses in the shade and avoiding vigorous activities during the hottest times of the day. These habits should be taught frequently, not only during heatwaves but throughout the hot months, to ensure that youngsters remain safe and healthy.

Vigilance applies to the social environment as well. In schools, daycare centers, and community settings, it is crucial that all staff members are taught to recognize and respond to heat-related illnesses. This joint responsibility ensures that children are protected even when they are not under the direct care of their parents. Schools and daycares should have clear heat safety policies in place, and staff should be authorized to take action if a kid displays signs of overheating.

One of the most crucial features of attentiveness is the capacity to respond swiftly and efficiently in an emergency. Knowing what to do if a youngster exhibits symptoms of heat exhaustion or heatstroke can save lives. This includes understanding when to seek medical care, how to cool the child down, and what procedures to take while waiting for emergency services to come. Parents and caregivers should familiarize themselves with basic first aid for heat-related diseases and ensure that they have access to emergency contact information at all times.

Vigilance also entails a broader knowledge of the social and economic elements that can enhance the risks associated with high heat. Families living in poverty or locations without appropriate green spaces or cooling facilities are at a higher risk. Recognizing these inequities and lobbying for resources and policies that address them is an important component of protecting vulnerable populations. Community activities, such as providing access to cooling centers, distributing fans, or offering financial support for air conditioning, can make a major difference in the lives of those most in danger.

Finally, vigilance involves staying educated about and participating in efforts to prevent the long-term implications of climate change, which is a significant driver of rising temperatures and more frequent heat waves. Supporting laws and efforts that reduce greenhouse gas emissions, promote renewable energy, and improve urban greenery can help safeguard future generations from the dangers of excessive heat. By being proactive and engaged in these broader efforts, individuals and communities can help establish a safer, healthier environment for all children.

In conclusion, protecting children from heat-related illnesses requires a consistent and watchful approach that combines education, preparation, and community involvement. By keeping children continually aware of the hazards, implementing preventative measures, and being prepared to respond promptly in an emergency, we can ensure that children are safe, healthy, and able to enjoy the summer months without fear of heat-related problems. The obligation is with all of us—parents, caregivers, educators, and community leaders—to create an atmosphere where children's health and well-being are valued, especially in the face of rising temperatures and changing climate conditions.

www.ingramcontent.com/pod-product-compliance
Lightning Source LLC
Chambersburg PA
CBHW070849250726
48662CB00003B/1438